Writing Patient/Client Notes

Ensuring Accuracy in Documentation

4th Edition

Writing Patient/Client Notes

Ensuring Accuracy in Documentation

4th Edition

Ginge Kettenbach, PhD, PT
Assistant Professor
Saint Louis University
St. Louis, Missouri

 F.A. Davis Company • Philadelphia

F. A. Davis Company
1915 Arch Street
Philadelphia, PA 19103
www.fadavis.com

Printed in the United States of America

Last digit indicates print number: 10 9 8 7 6 5 4 3 2

Acquisitions Editor: Melissa A. Duffield
Developmental Editor: Yvonne N. Gillam
Manager of Content Development: George W. Lang
Publisher: Margaret M. Biblis
Art and Design Manager: Carolyn O'Brien

As new scientific information becomes available through basic and clinical research, recommended treatments and drug therapies undergo changes. The author(s) and publisher have done everything possible to make this book accurate, up to date, and in accord with accepted standards at the time of publication. The author(s), editors, and publisher are not responsible for errors or omissions or for consequences from application of the book, and make no warranty, expressed or implied, in regard to the contents of the book. Any practice described in this book should be applied by the reader in accordance with professional standards of care used in regard to the unique circumstances that may apply in each situation. The reader is advised always to check product information (package inserts) for changes and new information regarding dose and contraindications before administering any drug. Caution is especially urged when using new or infrequently ordered drugs.

Library of Congress Cataloging-in-Publication Data

Kettenbach, Ginge.
Writing patient/client notes : ensuring accuracy in documentation / Ginge Kettenbach. — 4th ed.
   p. ; cm.
Rev. ed. of: Writing SOAP notes / Ginge Kettenbach. 3rd ed. c2004.
Includes bibliographical references.
ISBN-13: 978-0-8036-1878-7 (pbk. : alk. paper)
ISBN-10: 0-8036-1878-6 (pbk. : alk. paper)
1. Physical therapy—Documentation—Problems, exercises, etc. 2. Occupational therapy—Documentation—
Problems, exercises, etc. 3. Medical protocols—Problems, exercises, etc. 4. Note-taking—Problems, exercises,
etc. I. Kettenbach, Ginge. Writing SOAP notes. II. Title.
[DNLM: 1. Medical History Taking—Problems and Exercises. 2. Physical Therapy (Specialty)—Problems and
Exercises. 3. Physical Therapy Modalities—Problems and Exercises. 4. Writing—Problems and Exercises. WB
18.2 K43wa 2009]
RM701.6.K48 2009
615.8'2—dc22

                                                 2008030774

Foreword

Five years have passed since I last worked on a documentation textbook. At that time, the publication was *Writing SOAP Notes*. As always many things have happened in the health care environment that have influenced the revision of *Writing SOAP Notes* into this text. While the worksheets have stayed, more emphasis has been placed on the Patient/Client Management note and processes. This was done because SOAP notes are becoming less common and have become a method for poor documentation for some therapists. SOAP notes often do not show the therapist's unique thought processes and do not show justification for therapy.

Many parts of this workbook will look familiar to those who have used *Writing SOAP Notes* in the past. I decided to keep some form of SOAP note writing in this book for those who will still encounter SOAP notes in their clinical practice sites. If therapists used the form of SOAP note in this text that includes the patient/client management model, the SOAP note would not be problematic in documentation.

As with *Writing SOAP Notes*, this textbook assumes that the user has access to *The Guide to Physical Therapist Practice*. It is written as a book that teaches very new learners how to use the information in *The Guide to Physical Therapist Practice* for documentation purposes.

Books are never written or revised without help and support. I would like to thank the editors at F.A. Davis for their patience and support as I slowly worked on this project. My husband, Gerry, always encourages me to keep going with writing about documentation, although these projects always require sacrifices from him before I complete them. Without Gerry, this book would not exist. I would also like to thank my daughters, Kristen and Kathryn, who have grown up watching me write. They have now left home and still come back to help cover for me when I write and am too busy to do other things that need to be done in our lives. My final thanks go to my colleagues at Saint Louis University, particularly those who have contributed to this book. My colleagues in the Department of Health Informatics and Information Management have added three chapters about the medical record and reimbursement, areas in which they are the true experts. Theresa Bernsen, my physical therapy colleague, has written a chapter on where documentation will likely go in the future.

This book is written to help students learn about documentation. What every therapist does is very important and it is important that what they do is documented well. This book is only a small step in all of the things that must be learned to become a good therapist. It is my hope that it significantly contributes to the success of all therapists in their clinical practice.

Reviewers

Mary Dockter, PT, PhD
Assistant Professor and Director of Clinical Education
University of Mary
Department of Physical Therapy
Bismarck, ND

Lynda Jack, MS, PT
Assistant Professor of Physical Therapy
Florida Gulf Coast University
Department of Physical Therapy and Human
    Performance
Ft. Myers, FL

Jeffrey Komay, PTA
Instructor, ACCE
Western Technical College
Physical Therapist Assistant Department
Onalaska, WI

Carol A. Maritz, Ed.D, PT, GCS
Assistant Professor of Physical Therapy
University of the Sciences in Philadelphia
Department of Physical Therapy
Narberth, PA

Kimberly S. Peer, Ed.D, ATC, LAT
Athletic Training Education Program Coordinator,
    Associate Professor
Kent State University
Exercise, Leisure and Sport
Kent, OH

Susan E. Pivko, PT, DPT, Cert MDT
Assistant Professor, Director of Clinical Education
Hunter College
Department of Physical Therapy
New York, NY

Kelly Sass, MPT
Associate, Assistant Academic Coordinator of Clinical
    Education
University of Iowa
Graduate Prog in PT and Rehab Science
Iowa City, IA

Karen Wingert, DPT/RN
Clinical Associate Professor
University of Missouri
Department of Physical Therapy
Columbia, MO

Denise Wise, PhD, PT
Chair, Associate Professor
The College of St. Scholastica
Department of Physical Therapy
Duluth, MN

Benito J. Velasquez, DA, ATC, LAT
Associate Professor
University of Southern Mississippi
School of Human Performance and Recreation
Hattiesburg, MS

Contributors

Theresa G. Bernsen, PT, MA
Associate Professor
Saint Louis University
Doisy College of Health Sciences
Department of Physical Therapy
St. Louis, MO

Jeanne Donnelly, PhD, RHIA
Associate Professor
Department of Health Informatics and Information
   Management
Doisy College of Health Sciences
Saint Louis University
St. Louis, MO

Jody Smith, PhD, RHIA, FAHIMA
Department Chair and Professor
Department of Health Informatics and Information
   Management
Doisy College of Health Sciences
Saint Louis University
St. Louis, MO

Contents

How to Use This Book

This book was written to help new practitioners learn the skill of writing patient care notes. Like any other skill, writing notes takes practice. After each section of the note is discussed, an opportunity for practice is given in the worksheets at the end of the chapter. The chapters in Section I and several other chapters do not have worksheets because they cover prerequisite material needed for good documentation in general.

Abbreviations

Chapter 4, "Using Abbreviations," introduces you to the abbreviations most commonly seen and/or used by therapists. The abbreviations listed for Hospital XYZ are acceptable for use throughout the rest of the workbook. If an abbreviation does not appear on the list, it is not to be used to complete the worksheets.

Medical Terminology

Worksheets are offered after a very brief discussion of medical terminology. These worksheets serve only as a review of your knowledge of medical terminology. They assume that you have previously studied medical terminology in depth. If you cannot complete these worksheets without difficulty, a review of medical terminology is suggested.

Successful Completion of the Worksheets

The first chapters will further explain problem solving and both the SOAP and Patient/Client Management note formats and why patient care notes are written. A careful reading of the text in each chapter will assist you in successfully completing the worksheets and, ultimately, in successful note writing.

The benefits derived from completing the worksheets in this workbook depend upon the learner. If you are a novice at documentation, it is very important to complete each worksheet before referring to the answers in Appendix A. There are as many variations to note writing as there are practitioners. If your answers are not exactly the same as those provided, determine whether your answers would be considered acceptable and why the answers given in Appendix A might or might not be preferable to your answers. By first completing the worksheets and then comparing your work, you will learn in the same manner in which learning takes place in the clinic. Individual practice and feedback have always proved to be the best methods of learning to write notes. If you are an experienced therapist, the text should prove to be worthwhile; you can use the worksheets only as they prove to be of value to you.

Summary

The goal of this workbook is to provide the basic skills needed to document patient care. Appendices are provided for reference as you enter the clinic. A list of abbreviations to be used while completing the worksheets is included in Chapter 4. A review of medical terminology is provided in Chapter 3.

This book will not teach you to make all of the decisions necessary to examine, evaluate, and treat a patient. In each of the cases used in the worksheets, you will be given assistance in making decisions regarding setting goals or setting up an intervention plan. However, it is suggested that you take advantage of the examples of documentation of clinical decisions that are given to you as you complete the worksheets. In completing the worksheets, you are given the decisions, step by step, as they would be made by an experienced clinician. This is the type of clinical decision making that you will be expected to perform as you examine, evaluate, and treat patients while performing patient care as a professional.

I Background Information

Documentation is an important part of the care given to every patient.[1] Before a new professional can begin to write notes, some essential information is needed. This section provides the background information that is needed to begin the process of learning to document patient care.

Chapter 1 gives an overview of documentation and the differences and similarities between the two types of patient care notes presented in this text.

Chapter 2 discusses some important, basic guidelines that all practitioners should follow when writing in a medical record.

Chapter 3 is a review of medical terminology.

Chapter 4 discusses the use of abbreviations and provides an abbreviation list that will be used for all of the worksheets in this text.

The introduction, "How to Use This Book" on page—, is essential reading. Completing this book is an exercise that can be very useful, and this introductory material gives guidance on maximizing learning while using this text.

1 Introduction to Note Writing

Each day in the clinic, physical and occupational therapists, physical therapist assistants (PTAs), certified occupational therapy assistants (COTAs), and other health care professionals document patient care. One of the methods they use is a form of patient care note called a *SOAP Note*. Another method is the *Patient/Client Management Note*.

The SOAP and Patient/Client Management formats for writing notes are not the only methods used in therapy clinics. However, the SOAP format is commonly used throughout the country, and the Patient/Client Management format is being used by some clinicians as physical therapy practitioners become familiar with the *Guide to Physical Therapist Practice*.[1] It is rare for a health care professional not to encounter one of these two documentation formats, or a variation, during his or her career.

What SOAP Means

SOAP is an acronym. Each of the letters in SOAP stands for the name of a section of the patient note. The SOAP Note is divided as follows:

- **S** stands for *Subjective*.
- **O** stands for *Objective*.
- **A** stands for *Assessment*.
- **P** stands for *Plan*.

In most facilities, a fifth section, the *Problem,* is included before the S portion of the note.[2]

Components of the Patient/Client Management Note

The Patient/Client Management Model described in the *Guide to Physical Therapist Practice*[1] has the following components:

- History
- Systems Review
- Tests and Measures
- Evaluation
- Diagnosis
- Prognosis
- Plan of Care

The Purposes of Documentation

Documentation is an important role of therapists.[1] All health care professionals document their findings for several reasons, including the following:

1. Patient care notes record what the therapist does to manage the individual patient's case. These notes are placed in the patient's medical record. Patient care notes ensure that the rights of the therapist and the patient are protected legally should any question arise regarding the care provided to the patient. Patient care notes are considered legal documents, as are all parts of the medical record. In the event of litigation, the medical record may be subpoenaed, or the therapist may be called to testify in court or in a deposition on the contents of the medical record. The information in the patient care notes is recorded closer to the care given and may be more accurate than the therapist's memory.[3,4]

2. According to the *Guide to Physical Therapist Practice,* part of the role of the physical therapist is communication.[1] Good documentation is a method of communicating with all other health care professionals, including physicians, other therapists, and therapist assistants.[3] The patient care note communicates the results of the examination, the therapist's evaluation, the diagnosis, and the patient's prognosis. It communicates the therapist's (and patient's) expected outcomes and anticipated goals for the patient as well as the intervention plan, also known as the *Plan of Care.* The goal of such communication is to provide consistency and coordination among the services provided by various health care professionals.[1]

   A good patient care note can help a therapist communicate with other therapists or assistants who may provide substitute care for patients during the therapist's absence. The patient care note can be a helpful tool for communication between the therapist and assistant. In a rehabilitation center, school, or other setting using the rehabilitation team approach, the therapist's goals and the patient's level of function can be communicated to other professionals involved in the patient's care. Professionals providing services after the patient is discharged from one therapist's care may find the therapist's notes to be valuable in planning appropriate follow-up care.[1]

3. Part of the professional role of the physical therapist is advocacy.[1,5] Advocacy includes assisting the patient in obtaining insurance coverage for physical therapy by justifying the need for therapy services.[6] Third-party payers, such as Medicare reviewers and representatives from insurance companies, make decisions about reimbursement based on therapy notes.[7,8] These decisions can be greatly influenced by the quality and completeness of the note.[6–8]

4. Within the hospital and other types of facilities, documentation assists those who are making decisions regarding the patient's disposition and additional care needed after discharge from the facility.[9,10] Patient care notes written by the therapist or assistant may contribute significantly to discharge planning.[3]

5. Writing notes using either the SOAP Note or the Patient/Client Management Note format helps the therapist document his or her thought processes involved in patient care. By thinking in a structured manner with the use of evidence, the therapist can better make decisions regarding patient care. Thus, documentation is an excellent method of reflecting the structured clinical decision making of the therapist and problem solving of the assistant.[3,11]

6. Documentation of patient care can be used for quality assurance and improvement purposes. Standards that indicate and measure quality of care are established. Data can be gathered from the documented records of patient care and evaluated according to predetermined criteria. Results can be used for improving processes or for staff continuing education and professional development activities.[3,12]

7. Patient care notes can be used in outcomes research. As with quality assurance, certain criteria are initially set for the type of patient to be included and data to be gathered. Data from the notes can be assessed, and conclusions can be drawn about the types of interventions provided for patients with various diagnoses. This type of research is very critical for all health care professionals to ensure high-quality care in a cost-conscious atmosphere. To gather this information, it is vital that health care facilities and groups use a format that is consistent within their own facilities and with other health care entities. In this way, meaningful and statistically sound data can be compiled.[3,13–15]

8. Good documentation can help to educate others, including other health care professionals, third-party payors, and our patients, about the services that physical therapy can provide.[3,8,9] While the services we can provide seem obvious to us, they are not obvious to other people whom we contact every day during the practice of our profession.

9. Documentation can demonstrate compliance with federal, state, and local statutes and requirements. It can also assist with demonstrating compliance with requirements of accrediting agencies such as the Joint Commission on Accreditation of Healthcare Organizations (JCAHO) or the Commission on Accreditation of Rehabilitation Facilities (CARF).[3]

As a therapist or therapist assistant, it is important to realize that documentation is as integral to the patient care process as the examination, evaluation, or patient intervention. Each day a significant portion of time is spent by therapists and assistants in documenting what is done and why. Although it is true that the health care environment is demanding in terms of productivity and quality concerns, insufficient documentation can negatively affect patient care as much as an insufficient Plan of Care.[3]

Types of Notes

During the course of a patient's care, the patient is initially examined and evaluated, and the therapist generates a Diagnosis, Prognosis, and Plan of Care.[3] As the Plan of Care is implemented, the patient is re-examined and re-evaluated.[3,8,10,11] Finally, the patient is examined and evaluated on discharge from the therapist's care or when care is discontinued before the patient meets therapy goals.[1,10] Each of these examinations and evaluations is documented in a type of patient care note. An *initial note* is written after the first patient examination and evaluation and documents the Examination, Evaluation, Diagnosis, Prognosis, and Plan of Care.[3,10] A *progress note* is written periodically, reporting the results of re-examination and re-evaluation and changes in the Prognosis and Plan of Care, as needed.[3,10] A *discharge note* is written when therapy is discontinued or the patient is discharged from therapy, after a final examination and evaluation are performed. The discharge note addresses the results of the final examination and evaluation, the outcomes and goals achieved, a summary of the interventions received, and the final disposition of the patient.[3,10]

The Origin of SOAP Notes

The SOAP Note was introduced by Dr. Lawrence Weed as part of a system of organizing the medical record, called the problem-oriented medical record (POMR).[2,16–22] The POMR has one list of patient problems in the front of the chart, with each health care practitioner writing a separate SOAP Note to address each of the patient's problems. Many facilities never used the POMR; rather, they adopted a different organizational format for the medical record. Other facilities use an adapted POMR format. In any case, one contribution that clearly came from the POMR was the widespread use of the SOAP Note.

Professionals in many medical and health fields have adapted the original SOAP format of note writing into a practical tool that is used for documentation. Each field and each facility has its own variation and format for documentation. As you enter each clinical facility during your education and later during your professional practice, you will adapt your method of note writing to conform to the variation used by the facility. This workbook will teach you a comprehensive method of writing SOAP Notes that can be adapted to meet the requirements and needs of any facility.

The Patient/Client Management Note

The *Guide to Physical Therapist Practice* was initially published in 1997 and then revised in years thereafter.[1] After reading the framework for and description of practice published in the *Guide to Physical Therapist Practice*, physical therapists began to discuss the implications for documentation. Therapists attempted to construct documentation forms and computerized documentation formats that were consistent with this framework of practice.[15]

In the second edition of the *Guide to Physical Therapist Practice*, a Documentation Template was included for initial inpatient and outpatient settings.[1] Some facilities are fully adopting or adapting the Documentation Template for the Patient/Client Management Note. These facilities write patient care notes that use a format that contains all of the elements of the Patient/Client Management Model described in the *Guide to Physical Therapist Practice*. This workbook will teach you to write notes using the Patient/Client Management Note format. This format can be adapted to the needs of any facility.

The Patient/Client Management Process and Documentation Formats

As you approach the process of writing patient care notes, it is necessary to understand the relationship of the SOAP Note and the Patient/Client Management Note to the Patient/Client Management Process. This assists practitioners in determining where information is documented, no matter which note format is used.

The process of clinical decision making used by most therapists includes examining the patient, evaluating the data from the examination, formulating a diagnosis and prognosis, and determining the Plan of Care. Each of these processes is unique, and the results of each process must be documented in the medical record.[1,2,10]

Examination

The process of examination includes gathering information from the chart, other caregivers, the patient, the patient's family, caretakers, and friends. It also includes a systems review and tests and measures performed by the therapist.[1]

In the SOAP Note format, the information gathered in the examination is presented according to the nature of the *sources of information*. The information gathered from the medical record is usually written into an initial section of the note labeled the *Problem*. The information gathered from the patient and his or her family, caretakers, and friends is usually written into a section labeled the *Subjective (S)* section. Information gathered by the therapist performing a systems review and tests and measures is usually written into a section labeled the *Objective (O)* section.

In the Patient/Client Management Note format, the information gathered in the examination is recorded according to the *nature of the data*. The information gathered about the patient's history is included in a section labeled *History*.[1,3,10] The information gathered from performing a brief examination or screening of the patient's major systems addressed by physical therapy (cardiovascular, integumentary, musculoskeletal, and neuromuscular) is written into a section labeled the *Systems Review*. Information gathered from a brief screening of the patient's communication, affect, cognition, learning style, and education needs is also written into the Systems Review section of the note.[1,3,10] Results from specific tests and measures performed by the therapist are documented in a section of the note labeled *Tests and Measures*.[1,3,10]

Evaluation

The evaluation process includes a synthesis and discussion of the clinical findings, usually presented in the form of a problem list and/or discussion of factors influencing the patient's condition or progress in therapy. This is the section of the notes in which the therapist's clinical decision-making processes are evident.[1] In the Patient/Client Management Note format, this information is presented in the Evaluation part of the note.[3,10] A discussion of other health care professionals to which the therapist has referred the patient or believes the patient should be referred is included in this section, along with the reasons for referral. The *Guide to Physical Therapist Practice* further defines the process of evaluation.[1]

In the SOAP Note format, this information appears in the section labeled *Assessment (A)*. The information

is written as part of the subsections under "A" labeled *Evaluation*.

Diagnosis

The Diagnosis section of the note includes a discussion of the relationship of the patient's functional deficits to the patient's impairments. If appropriate, a discussion of the relationship of the patient's disability to functional deficits and impairments can be discussed. The patient can be placed in a diagnostic category as well as in one or more of the practice patterns listed in the *Guide to Physical Therapist Practice*. If more than one practice pattern is applicable, the therapist indicates which practice pattern is primary. A discussion of the relevant functional deficits and impairments indicating the relevant practice pattern or patterns may occur in this section. An ICD9-CM label can be listed. Other diagnostic labels can be used, as indicated by evidence. The *Guide to Physical Therapist Practice* further defines the process of diagnosis performed by physical therapists.[1]

In the SOAP Note, the diagnosis is recorded in the A section of the note in a subsection labeled Diagnosis. The contents of the subsection are identical to the contents listed for the Patient/Client Management Note.

Prognosis

The Prognosis section of the note in physical therapy includes the predicted level of improvement that the patient will be able to achieve and the predicted amount of time to achieve that level of improvement. This section should also include the therapist's professional opinion of the patient's rehabilitation potential. Plans for discharge and discontinuation of therapy may be listed in this subsection of the note. Future therapy that the therapist believes will be needed after discontinuing care from the therapist's practice setting can be discussed in this section of the note, including the proposed duration of future therapy.[1] Projected final outcomes of therapy can be stated in functional terms, if not listed in the Expected Outcomes part of the Plan of Care.[3]

In the SOAP Note, a discussion of the prognosis and the rationale for the prognosis is recorded in the A section of the note in a subsection labeled Prognosis.

Plan of Care

The Plan of Care includes the Expected Outcomes (Long-Term Goals), Anticipated Goals (Short-Term Goals), and Interventions, including an Education Plan for the patient or the patient's caregivers or significant others.[1] Some facilities may include the Plan of Care with the Prognosis in the note. In both note formats, this information is recorded in a section entitled *Plan of Care (P)*.

Documentation of Health-Care Delivery by the Physical Therapist Assistant or Occupational Therapy Assistant

The PTA or COTA reads the initial documentation of the Examination, Evaluation, Diagnosis, Prognosis, Expected Outcomes, Anticipated Goals, and Intervention Plan, and is expected to follow the Plan of Care as outlined by the therapist in the initial patient note. After the patient has been seen by the PTA or COTA for a time (the time varies according to the policies of each facility or health care system and state law), the PTA or COTA must write a progress note documenting any measurements of change in the patient's status that have occurred since the therapist's initial note was written. Also, after discussion with the therapist concerning the Diagnosis, Prognosis, Expected Outcomes, Anticipated Goals, and Interventions, the assistant may rewrite or respond to the previously written anticipated goals and document a revised Plan of Care accordingly. In many facilities, the therapist then cosigns the assistant's notes, indicating agreement with what is documented in the notes. (Once again, this depends on the facility's policies and state law.) It is always the responsibility of the therapist to make changes in the Plan of Care through the process of evaluation and the revision of anticipated goals.[1]

It is extremely important for both therapists and assistants to remember the importance of the role of assistants in documenting patient care. Assistants can develop the skill to participate as fully in documentation of patient care as they do in delivering patient care. With health care delivery continually changing, assisting with documentation is a valuable role for the assistant, and documentation skills are as crucial to the assistant as they are to the therapist. Therefore, PTA and COTA students are encouraged to take full advantage of the skills to be learned from this workbook.

Some of the notes written in the worksheets are examples of initial patient care notes. Although it is acknowledged that the assistant does not write an initial note in the clinic, the same skills used to write initial notes are used to write progress notes after discussion with the therapist. Therefore, assistant students are encouraged to take advantage of the opportunities to write all of the sample notes in all of the worksheets. If it is helpful, think of the examples of initial notes as progress notes during which the therapist and assistant worked together to perform certain patient examinations and discussed the Evaluation, Diagnosis, Prognosis, and revision of the Anticipated goals and Interventions in the Plan of Care. Each facility differs in its use of assistants in both occupational and physical therapy. However, no matter what the specific details of the assistant's role, it is clear that assistants need good documentation skills.

Summary and Objective

This workbook will teach you to write two types of documentation, both the Patient/Client Management Note and the SOAP Note. Both note formats allow the documentation of patient care and both follow the Patient/Client Management Process described in the *Guide to Physical Therapist Practice*.[1]

The Patient/Client Management Note and the SOAP Note include the same information. The information is organized differently in each note format, particularly in the way the examination of the patient is documented. The information from the Evaluation, Diagnosis, Prognosis and Plan of Care sections is organized similarly in the two note formats. Appendix B has a chart summarizing the information in the Patient/Client Management Process and the manner in which it is documented in each note format.

Documentation has many purposes, including ensuring quality care, communication, and discharge planning. Documentation has become very important in a health care atmosphere that includes litigation, the need of third-party payors to obtain clear and accurate information, and the need for research on the outcomes of the interventions used in rehabilitation. Both methods of writing notes serve as guides and reflect clinical decision making, demonstrating accountability and justification for quality patient care, and documenting patient care.

References

1. American Physical Therapy Association: Guide to Physical Therapist Practice, ed. 2, and CD-ROM. American Physical Therapy Association, Alexandria, VA, 2003.
2. Feitelberg, SB: The Problem Oriented Record System in Physical Therapy. University of Vermont, Burlington, VT, 1975.
3. American Physical Therapy Association: Defensible Documentation for Patient/Client Management. Accessed at http://www.apta.org/AM/Template. cfm?Section=Documentation4&Template=/MembersOnly. cfm&ContentID=37776 on March 9, 2007.
4. Kolber, M, and Lucado, AM.: Risk management strategies in physical therapy: documentation to avoid malpractice. International Journal of Health Care Quality Assurance 18(2):123–129, 2005.
5. Professionalism in Physical Therapy: Core Values. Accessed at http://www.apta.org/AM/Template.cfm?Section= Professionalism1&CONTENTID=35254&TEMPLATE=/ CM/ContentDisplay.cfm on March 9, 2007.
6. Schaum, K: New 2006 physical therapy cap and exception process. Advances in Skin and Wound Care 19(5):251–256, 2006.

7. Smith, R: Rehab economics: private practice keeps on truckin'. Rehab Management 14(5):70–74, 2001.

8. Babb, R: Documentation and reimbursement strategies in aquatic physical therapy. Journal of Aquatic Physical Therapy 8(2):33–36, 2000.

9. American Physical Therapy Association: APTA Guide for Professional Conduct. Accessed at http://www.apta.org/ AM/Template.cfm?Section= Policies_and_ Bylaws&Template=/CM/HTMLDisplay. cfm&ContentID=24781 on March 9, 2007.

10. American Physical Therapy Association: Guidelines: Physical Therapy Documentation Of Patient/Client Management. Accessed at http://www.apta.org/AM/Template. cfm?Section=Home&TEMPLATE=/CM/ ContentDisplay. cfm&CONTENTID=31688 on March 9, 2007.

11. Rothstein, JM, Echternach, JL, and Riddle, DL: The Hypothesis-Oriented Algorithm for Clinicians II (HOAC II): A guide for patient management. Physical Therapy 83(5):455–470, 2003.

12. Brown, J: When was the last time you reviewed your hospital outpatient chart review program? Twelve key criteria you should use during the evaluation process. Journal of Health Care Compliance 6(5):36–40, 2004.

13. Guccione, A, et al: Development and testing of a self-report instrument to measure actions: Outpatient Physical Therapy Improvement in Movement Assessment Log (OPTIMAL). Physical Therapy 85(6):515–530, 2005.

14. Waldrop, S: APTA Connect: Software for improved documentation and outcomes measurement. PT—Magazine of Physical Therapy 14(10):54, 82, 2006.

15. Reynolds, JP: To compare apples with apples: guide-based documentation. PT—Magazine of Physical Therapy 6(6):60–2, 64, 66–71, 1998.

16. Berni, R, and Ready, H: Problem-Oriented Medical Record Implementation. Allied Health Peer Review. Mosby, St. Louis, 1978.

17. Hill, JR: The Problem-Oriented Approach to Physical Therapy Care. American Physical Therapy Association, Washington, DC, 1977.

18. Hurst, JW, and Walker, HK (eds): The Problem-Oriented System. Medcom Press, 1972.

19. Wakefield, JS, and Yarnall, SR (eds): Implementing the Problem-Orienting Medical Record, MCSA, Seattle, WA, 1976.

20. Weed, LL: Medical Records, Medical Education, and Patient Care. Year Book Medical Publishers, Inc., Chicago, IL, 1971.

21. Weed LL. Medical records that guide and teach. New England Journal of Medicine. 278(11):593–600, 1968.

22. Weed, LL: Medical Records, Patient care and medical education. Irish Journal of Medical Science 17:271–282, 1964.

2 Writing in a Medical Record

*T*he writing style used in patient care notes at most clinical facilities differs from the style most students are accustomed to using when writing papers, reports, and academic assignments. Writing in patient charts or files requires using medical abbreviations and terminology, and emphasizes brevity. The following guidelines are provided to assist you in becoming accustomed to writing in a medical record.

Accuracy

Never record falsely, exaggerate, guess at, or make up data.[1] Patient care notes are parts of a permanent, legal document called the *medical record*.[1,2] Incorrect spelling, grammar, and punctuation can be misleading. All information should be stated in a factual manner. Criticisms of other staff members, colleagues, or the patient, or complaints about working conditions should not be included in the patient care note. The note is about the patient's condition, not about the health care provider or the health care provider's reactions to other people.

Brevity

Information should be stated concisely. Use short, succinct sentences. Avoid long-winded statements. Also avoid strings of short clauses connected by "and." It is permissible to use sentence fragments or outline form at some facilities. Whatever style is used, it is important to be consistent in style to avoid confusion and to comply with the policies of the facility or practice setting. If a flow sheet or table of information is used for the results of tests and measures, additional information demonstrating the therapist's clinical judgment must be documented in addition to the table of information.[2]

Abbreviations can help with brevity. However, too many abbreviations can make a document almost impossible to use. Abbreviations used in documentation should be from a list accepted at the facility at which you practice and should be the more standard abbreviations that you have encountered throughout your clinical practice experience.[1,2] During your orientation to the facility, you should ask for a copy of that facility's standard list of abbreviations. This list of abbreviations should be attached to any documentation that is sent outside of your facility, including third-party payors.

| example |

Brief: Pt. amb. 10 ft. in parallel bars indep. but required min. assist of 1 to turn around in parallel bars; Pt. did not have the balance to turn unsupported and needed instruction as well. Sit↔stand from w/c indep. using parallel bars for support.

Longwinded: Once the patient wheeled up to the parallel bars and positioned himself in front of the parallel bars, he locked his w/c, raised the foot plates, and scooted forward from the seat of the chair. He then gripped the parallel bars with his hands and on the count of 3 was able to pull himself up to a standing position without any assistance from the therapist. Once standing, he was able to ambulate by positioning his arms forward and then taking steps. He could lead with either right or left foot. Upon turning in the parallel bars, he was unable to let go with one arm to pivot his body around. Therapist had to give some support until the patient was turned around and both arms were back on the parallel bars.

Brevity can also be overdone. Documentation should include information to describe the patient/client care that has occurred. Almost every statement in the medical record contains a verb (or some sort of punctuation to replace a verb; see *Punctuation*, below).

Clarity

The wording of all patient care notes should be such that the meaning is immediately clear to the reader. Sudden shifts in tense from past to present should be avoided.

| example |

Incorrect: Pt stated she lived alone. Describes 5 steps s̄ hand railing at entry of her 1-story house. Denied previous use of assist. device.

Correct: States lives alone. Describes 5 steps s̄ hand railing at entry of her 1-story house. Denies previous use of assist. device.

Avoid vague terminology.

Vague: ROM is ↑.

Vague: Pt. is feeling better.

Vague: Amb. c̄ some assist.

Clear: Ⓡ shoulder flexion AROM is ↑ to 0–70°

Clear: Pt. states she knows she is feeling better, indicated by her ability to perform light house-keeping tasks for 2 hrs. ā tiring.

Clear: Pt. amb. c̄ walker NWB Ⓛ LE for ~20 ft. × 2 c̄ min. +1 assist.

Using abbreviations that are standard to the facility is absolutely essential to ensure clarity in note writing. Terminology used within a rehabilitation department or practice, such as *minimal assistance*, or *min assist*, should be well defined and used in a consistent manner by all therapists in the department or practice.

Examples of Errors in Accuracy, Brevity, and Clarity

INCORRECT: Pt. was unable to perform activity due to *muscle absence.* (inaccurate and unclear)

CORRECT: ... due to *muscle paralysis.*

INCORRECT: *Watch for* return of *absent muscles.* (unclear and inaccurate)

CORRECT: *Re-examine* prn for *motor return.*

INCORRECT: Pt. is *sore.* (too brief; unclear)

CORRECT: Pt. is *hypersensitive to touch.*

INCORRECT: Pt. *didn't have any tightness.* (wordy; unclear)

CORRECT: *No ROM limitations* noted.

INCORRECT: Had his Ⓡ leg *cut off because of circulation problems.* (wordy)

CORRECT: Ⓡ transtibial *amputation 2° to PVD.*

INCORRECT: Pt. was unable to wiggle toes *when asked to.* (wordy)

CORRECT: Pt. was unable to wiggle toes *upon request.*

INCORRECT: Examination *was* incomplete *because of* pt. confusion. (wordy and unclear)

CORRECT: Examination incomplete *2° to* Pt's inability to follow commands.

Punctuation

Hyphen (-)

Hyphens should be avoided in notes because they can be confused with the minus signs used in muscle grades or negatives (as in SLR: – on Ⓡ ; one exception is the common use of a hyphen instead of the word through or to (as in AROM Ⓡ knee: 0–48°).

Semicolon (;)

Instead of overusing "states" in the subjective part of the note, a semicolon can be used to connect two related statements.

Wordy: States position of comfort for sleep is on Ⓡ side. States pain does not awaken Pt. at night.

Brief: States position of comfort for sleep is on Ⓡ side; pain does not awaken Pt. at night.

Colon (:)

A colon can be used instead of "is."

Wordy: AROM Ⓡ shoulder flexion is 0–90°.

Brief: AROM Ⓡ shoulder flexion: 0–90°.

Correcting Errors

Correction fluid or tape should *not* be used on a medical record. Trying to destroy or attempting to obliterate information makes it look as if the health professional is trying to "cover up" malpractice. The proper method of correcting a charting mistake while writing a patient care note is to put a line through the error, write the date, and initial above the error.

                    VKK 2/28/08

Correct: ~~some~~ min +1 assist.

Signing Your Notes

You should sign every entry that you make into the medical record. The process of signing patient care notes is called *authentication.*[1,2] All notes should be signed with your legal signature (your last name and legal first name or initials). No nicknames should be used. Initials should follow your name indicating your status as a therapist or therapist assistant.

Sue Brown, PT or James Smith, PTA
Maryann Jones, OTR or B.J. McDonald, COTA

In some facilities, there is a custom of using additional initials (L, P, or R) prior to PT or PTA. In some states, state law dictates certain letters follow a therapist's signature. If state law allows, the American Physical Therapy Association advocates the use of PT or PTA only. The American Occupational Association advocates the use of OTR or COTA. In some clinics, students sign their notes SPT or SPTA, OTS or OTAS. In others, students are required to sign their name only. In either case, the signature of a student should always be followed by a slash and then the signature of the supervising therapist.

> **example**
>
> Gene White, SPT/Sue Brown, PT
> Peter Maxwell, OTS/Maryann Jones, OTR

Referring to Yourself

Notes discuss the patient, not the therapist.

> **example**
>
> **Incorrect:** I helped this patient transfer c̄ min assist. from his w/c to the plinth.
>
> **Correct:** Pt. transferred w/c↔plinth c̄ min. assist. to compensate for balance issues.

If for some reason a therapist must make reference to himself or herself, most facilities prefer that the reference be made in the third person as *therapist, physical therapist,* or *occupational therapist.*

> **example**
>
> Pt. states therapist should be putting his shoes on for him like his family does at home.

Blank or Empty Lines

Empty lines should not be left between one entry and another, nor should empty lines be left within a single entry.[1] Empty lines are areas in which another person could falsify information already charted. Adding even one word, such as *not,* to a note can completely change the meaning of the note's content.

Writing Orders in a Chart

When a physician gives an order to a therapist, the therapist is the professional responsible for writing it in the chart. When beginning at a new facility, it is important to ask about the procedure used for verbal orders. In writing an order in the chart, the following format is standard in most facilities:

date/time/order
v.o. physician's name/therapist's signature, OTR (or PT)

> **example**
>
> 12-24-2008/10:50/Pt. may be FWB in PT.
> v.o. Dr. Ache/Sue Brown, PT

Once the order is written by the therapist in the chart, the physician cosigns the order the next time he or she sees the medical record or as soon as possible thereafter.

Summary and Objective

Writing in a medical record should be brief, accurate, and clear. Errors should be corrected, *not* erased or covered with correction fluid. You should use your legal signature as you would on any legal document. If you follow the guidelines in this chapter and apply them throughout the exercises in this book, you will develop a good medical writing style that you will use daily in clinical practice.

References

1. Kolber, M, and Lucado, AM: Risk management strategies in physical therapy: documentation to avoid malpractice. International Journal of Health Care Quality assurance 18(2):123–129, 2005.

2. Defensible Documentation for Patient/Client Management. Accessed at http://www.apta.org/AM/Template. cfm?Section=Documentation4&Template=/MembersOnly. cfm&ContentID=37776 on March 9, 2007.

3 | Medical Terminology

*B*efore any health care professional can begin reading or writing medical documentation in an acceptable manner, she or he must be familiar with the terminology commonly used in medical writing. Most of the terms have Greek- or Latin-based prefixes, suffixes, or roots. It is often easy to ascertain the meaning of a particular term if the more commonly used prefixes, suffixes, and roots are known.

Learning medical terminology and its prefixes, suffixes, and roots is outside the scope of this workbook. Some basic knowledge of medical terminology is assumed.

The worksheets should serve as a review of medical terminology. The terms used in these worksheets are encountered frequently by therapists and assistants. If you are unfamiliar with the terms and definitions used in these worksheets, it is suggested that you review medical terminology before continuing in this workbook.

term = prefix + *root*	*Example:* Sclero*derma*
OR	
term = *root* + suffix	*Example: Osteo*porosis
OR	
term = prefix + *root* + suffix	*Example:* Syn*dactyl*ism[1]

Reference

1. Gylys, BA, and Masters, RM: Medical Terminology: A Systems Approach, ed 3. F.A. Davis Company, Philadephia, 2007.

Medical Terminology

> ■ **PART I.** Write the appropriate term for the definition.

1. Tumor of the bone _____

2. Abnormally low blood sugar _____

3. Beneath the skin _____

4. Above the symphysis pubis _____

5. Pertaining to the back of the body _____

6. Toward the head _____

7. Abnormal redness of the skin _____

8. Between the ribs _____

9. Front of the body _____ or

_____

10. Conducting toward a structure _____

> **PART II.** Write the appropriate definition for the term listed.

1. Symphysis pubis _____
   _____

2. Cardiomegaly _____
   _____

3. Meniscectomy _____
   _____

4. Chondroma _____
   _____

5. Arthrodesis _____
   _____

6. Craniotomy _____
   _____

7. Neurology _____
   _____

8. Anesthesia _____
   _____

9. Phlebitis _____
   _____

10. Hypertension _____
    _____

Answers to "Medical Terminology: Worksheet 1" are provided in Appendix A.

Medical Terminology

> **PART I.** Write the appropriate term for the definition.

1. Joint inflammation   _____

2. Inspection of joint with a scope _____

3. Disease of a muscle   _____

4. Difficult or bad breathing   _____

5. Lack of coordination   _____

6. Softening of cartilage   _____

7. Inflammation of the brain   _____

8. Tumor of the meninges   _____

9. Paralysis of one half of the body _____

10. Beneath the clavicle   _____

PART II. Write the appropriate definition for the term listed.

1. Analgesia _____

_____

2. Bilateral _____

_____

3. Contralateral _____

_____

4. Aphasia _____

_____

5. Tendinitis _____

_____

6. Bradykinesia _____

_____

7. Dysphagia _____

_____

8. Arthralgia _____

_____

9. Cerebromalacia _____

_____

10. Costochondral _____

_____

Answers to "Medical Terminology: Worksheet 2" are provided in Appendix A.

4 | Using Abbreviations

Abbreviations are used to save time and space while writing notes. To ensure that everyone involved in the patient's care can understand what others have written in the medical record, most medical facilities have a list of approved abbreviations, and these are the only abbreviations that should be used in that particular facility.[1,2] A committee at each facility approves this list. The list of acceptable abbreviations varies from one facility to the next.

The list of abbreviations that follows will be used as the approved list for all of the worksheets in this book. Any abbreviations not on this list are considered unacceptable for these worksheets. When you begin your career, please remember that the list of acceptable abbreviations for your clinical facility must be used. During orientation to any clinical facility in which you practice, you should ask about the location of the approved abbreviations list and become particularly familiar with the abbreviations used frequently by the facility.

Approved Abbreviations and Symbols for Hospital XYZ[3,4]

A:	assessment
ABI	acquired brain injury
afib	atrial fibrillation
A-line	arterial line
A-V	arteriovenous
AAA	abdominal aortic aneurysm
AAROM	active assistive range of motion
Abd or abd	abduction
ABG	arterial blood gases
ac	before meals
AC joint	acromioclavicular joint
ACL	anterior cruciate ligament
ACTH	adrenocorticotrophic hormone
Add or add	adduction
ADL	activities of daily living
ad lib	at discretion
adm	admission, admitted
AE	above elbow
AFO	ankle foot orthosis
AIDS	acquired immune deficiency syndrome
AIIS	anterior inferior iliac spine
AJ	ankle jerk
AK	above knee
ALS	amyotrophic lateral sclerosis

a.m.	morning
AMA	against medical advice
amb	ambulation, ambulating, ambulated, ambulate, ambulates
ANS	autonomic nervous system
ant	anterior
AP	anterior-posterior
ARDS	adult respiratory distress syndrome
ARF	acute renal failure
AROM	active range of motion
ASA	aspirin
ASAP or asap	as soon as possible
ASCVD	arteriosclerotic cardiovascular disease
ASHD	arteriosclerotic heart disease
ASIS	anterior superior iliac spine
assist.	assistance, assistive
AVM	arteriovenous malformation
B/S	bedside
BBB	bundle branch block
BE	below elbow
BID or bid	twice a day
bilat. or B	bilateral, bilaterally
BK	below knee
BM	bowel movement
BOS	base of support
BP	blood pressure
bpm	beats per minute
BR	bedrest
BRP	bathroom privileges
BS	breath sounds or bowel sounds
BUN	blood urea nitrogen (blood test)
C	centigrade
C&S	culture and sensitivity
c/o	complains of
CA	cancer, carcinoma
CABG	coronary artery bypass graft
CAD	coronary artery disease
cal	calories
CAT	computerized axial tomography
CBC	complete blood cell (count)
CC, C/C	chief complaint
CF	cystic fibrosis
CHF	congestive heart failure
cm	centimeter
CMV	cytomegalovirus
CNS	central nervous system
CO	cardiac output
CO$_2$	carbon dioxide

cont.	continue
COPD	chronic obstructive pulmonary disease
COTA	certified occupational therapy assistant
CP	cerebral palsy
CPAP	continuous positive airway pressure
CPR	cardiopulmonary resuscitation
CRF	chronic renal failure
CSF	cerebrospinal fluid
CV	cardiovascular
CWI	crutch walking instructions
CXR	chest x-ray
Cysto	cystoscopic examination
D/C	discontinued or discharged
dept.	department
DIP	distal interphalangeal (joint)
DJD	degenerative joint disease
DM	diabetes mellitus
DNR	do not resuscitate
DO	doctor of osteopathy
DOB	date of birth
DOE	dyspnea on exertion
DTR	deep tendon reflex
DVT	deep vein thrombosis
Dx	diagnosis
ECF	extended care facility
ECG, EKG	electrocardiogram
ED	emergency department
EEG	electroencephalogram
EENT	ear, eyes, nose, throat
EMG	electromyogram, electromyography
E.R.	emergency room
eval.	evaluation
ext.	extension
FBS	fasting blood sugar
FEV	forced expiratory volume
FH	family history
flex	flexion
FRC	functional residual capacity
ft.	foot, feet (the measurement, not the body part)
FUO	fever of unknown origin
FVC	forced vital capacity
FWB	full weight bearing
fx	fracture
GB	gallbladder
GI	gastrointestinal
g	gram
GSW	gunshot wound
GYN	gynecology
h, hr.	hour
H&H, H/H	hematocrit and hemoglobin
H&P	history and physical
h/o	history of
HA, H/A	headache
Hb, Hgb	hemoglobin
Hct	hematocrit

HCVD	hypertensive cardiovascular disease
HEENT	head, ear, eyes, nose, throat
HEP	home exercise program
HIV	human immunodeficiency virus
HNP	herniated nucleus pulposus
HOB	head of bed
HR	heart rate
hs	at bedtime
ht.	height
Ht	hematocrit
Htn or HTN	hypertension
Hx	history
I&O	intake and output
IADL	instrumental activities of daily living
ICU	intensive care unit
IDDM	insulin-dependent diabetes mellitus
IM	intramuscular
imp.	impression
in.	inches
indep	independent
IMV	intermittent mandatory ventilation
inf	inferior
IRDS	infant respiratory distress syndrome
IS	incentive spirometry
IV	intravenous
KAFO	knee-ankle-foot orthosis
kcal	kilocalories
kg	kilogram
KJ	knee jerk
KUB	kidney, ureter, bladder
L or l.	liter
L	left
lat	lateral
lb.	pound
LBBB	left bundle branch block
LBP	low back pain
LE	lower extremity
LOC	loss of consciousness, level of consciousness
LMN	lower motor neuron
LOS	length of stay
LP	lumbar puncture
m	meter
MAP	mean arterial pressure
max	maximal
MD	medical doctor; doctor of medicine
MED	minimal erythemal dose
Meds.	medications
mg	milligram
MI	myocardial infarction
min	minimal
min.	minute
ml	milliliter
mm	millimeter
MMT	manual muscle test
mo.	month

mod	moderate		**prn**	whenever necessary, as often as necessary
MP, MEP	metacarpophalangeal		**PROM**	passive range of motion
MRSA	methicillin-resistant *Staphylococcus aureus*		**PSIS**	posterior-superior iliac spine
MVA	motor vehicle accident		**PT**	physical therapy, physical therapist (used after therapist's signature)
NDT	neurodevelopmental treatment		**PT/PTT**	prothrombin time/partial thrombo-plastin time
neg.	negative			
NG or ng	nasogastric		**Pt., pt.**	patient
N.H.	nursing home		**PTA**	physical therapist assistant
NIDDM	non–insulin-dependent diabetes mellitus		**PTA**	prior to admission
nn	nerve		**PTB**	patellar tendon bearing
noc	night, at night		**PVD**	peripheral vascular disease
NPO or npo	nothing by mouth		**PWB**	partial weight bearing
NSR	normal sinus rhythm		**q**	every
NWB	non–weight bearing		**qid**	four times a day
O:	objective		**qh**	every hour
OA	osteoarthritis		**qn**	every night
OB	obstetrics		**qt.**	quart
OBS	organic brain syndrome		**R**	right
od	once daily		**RA**	rheumatoid arthritis
OOB	out of bed		**RBBB**	right bundle branch block
O.P.	outpatient		**RBC**	red blood cell (count)
O.R.	operating room		**R.D.**	registered dietician
ORIF	open reduction, internal fixation		**re:**	regarding
OT	occupational therapy, occupational therapist		**rehab**	rehabilitation
			reps	repetitions
OTR	occupational therapist (used to follow official signature of the occupational therapist)		**resp**	respiratory, respiration
			RN	registered nurse
			R/O or r/o	rule out
oz.	ounce		**ROM**	range of motion
P	poor		**ROS**	review of systems
P:	plan, intervention plan, plan of care		**RR**	respiratory rate
P.A.	physician's assistant		**RROM**	resistive range of motion
PA	posterior/anterior		**RT**	respiratory therapist, respiratory therapy
para	paraplegia		**Rx**	intervention plan, prescription, therapy
pc	after meals		**SACH**	solid ankle cushion heel
PCL	posterior cruciate ligament		**SCI**	spinal cord injury
PE	pulmonary embolus		**SC joint**	sternoclavicular joint
PEEP	positive end expiratory pressure		**sec.**	seconds
per	by/through		**SED**	suberythemal dose
p.o.	by mouth		**sig**	directions for use, give as follows, let it be labeled
PERRLA	pupils equal, round, reactive to light, and accommodation			
			SI(J)	sacroiliac (joint)
P.H.	past history		**SLE**	systemic lupus erythematosus
p.m.	afternoon		**SLP**	speech-language pathologist
PMH	past medical history		**SLR**	straight leg raise
PNF	proprioceptive neuromuscular facilitation		**SNF**	skilled nursing facility
			SOAP	subjective, objective, assessment, plan
PNI	peripheral nerve injury		**SOB**	shortness of breath
POMR	problem-oriented medical record		**S/P**	status post (e.g., "S/P hip fx" means "Pt. fx her hip in the recent past.")
pos.	positive			
poss	possible		**spec**	specimen
post	posterior		**stat.**	immediately, at once
post-op	after surgery (operation)		**sup**	superior
PRE	progressive-resistive exercise		**Sx**	symptoms
pre-op	before surgery (operation)		**tab**	tablet

TB	tuberculosis		**yd.**	yard
TBI	traumatic brain injury		**yr.**	year
tbsp.	tablespoon		**+1 (+2, etc.)**	assistance (assistance of 1 person given; also written "assistance of 1." Examples: amb ... c̄ min + 1 assist., or amb ... c̄ +1 min assist., or amb ... c̄ min assist. of 1)
TENS, TNS	transcutaneous electrical nerve stimulator/stimulation			
THA	total hip arthroplasty			
ther ex	therapeutic exercise			
TIA	transient ischemic attack		♂	male
tid	three times daily		♀	female
TKA	total knee arthroplasty		↓	down, downward, decrease, diminished
TM(J)	temporomandibular (joint)		↑	up, upward, increase, augmented
TNR	tonic neck reflex (also ATNR, STNR)		//	parallel or parallel bars (also written "// bars")
t.o.	telephone order			
TPR	temperature, pulse, and respiration		c̄	with
tsp.	teaspoon		s̄	without
TUR/TURP	transurethral resection		p̄	after
Tx	traction		ā	before
TV	tidal volume		~ or ≈	approximately
UA	urine analysis		Δ	change
UE	upper extremity		=	equal
UMN	upper motor neuron		+ or (+)	plus, positive (positive also abbreviated "pos.")
URI	upper respiratory infection			
US	ultrasound		− or (−)	minus, negative (negative also abbreviated "neg.")
UTI	urinary tract infection			
UV	ultraviolet		#	number (#1 = number 1), pounds (5# wt. = 5 pound weight; *pound* also abbreviated "lbs.")
VC	vital capacity			
VD	venereal disease			
v.o. or VO	verbal orders (e.g., v.o. Dr. Smith/ assistant's signature)		/	per
			%	percent
vol.	volume		+, &, et.	and
v.s.	vital signs		↔	to and from
w/c	wheelchair		→	to progressing toward, approaching
W/cm²	watts per square centimeter		1°	primary
WBC	white blood cell (count)		2°	secondary, secondary to
wk.	week			
WNL	within normal limits			
wt.	weight			
×	number of times performed (e.g., ×2 is twice; ×3 is 3 times)			
y/o or y.o.	years old			

Using Abbreviations: Examples

The following are examples of the use of abbreviations in medical records.

1. In the physician's notes, you may find the following: Pt. has hx of Htn, ASHD, CHF, MI in 2005, TIA in 2006.	<u>Translation:</u> The patient has a history of hypertension, arteriosclerotic heart disease, congestive heart failure, myocardial infarction in 2005, transient ischemic attack in 2006.
2. Orders written in the chart: Up ad lib ASA q 4 hr. BRP prn NPO p̄ midnight v.o. Dr. Smith/Janice Jones, OTR	<u>Translation:</u> Up at discretion (patient's discretion) Aspirin every 4 hours Bathroom privileges when necessary Nothing by mouth after midnight Verbal order given by Dr. Smith to Janice Jones, occupational therapist
3. In PT note: Rx: AROM Ⓡ ankle bid	<u>Translation:</u> Treatment intervention: Active range of motion right ankle two times per day.
4. In chart in doctor's initial note: imp: COPD; R/O lung CA	<u>Translation:</u> Impression: Chronic obstructive pulmonary disease; rule out lung cancer.
5. Physician's orders: Record I&O; all meds per IV; NPO; transfer Pt. to ICU	<u>Translation:</u> Record intake and output. All medications through intravenous tube. Nothing by mouth. Transfer patient to the intensive care unit.

Summary and Objective

You will be expected to be able to both interpret and use abbreviations in the medical record. You will encounter most of the abbreviations listed in this chapter when you practice in the clinic. Any time you write a note, you will be expected to use abbreviations properly.

References

1. Defensible Documentation for Patient/Client Management. Accessed at http://www.apta.org/AM/Template.cfm?Section=Documentation4&Template=/MembersOnly.cfm&ContentID=37776 on March 9, 2007.
2. Kolber, M, and Lucado, AM: Risk management strategies in physical therapy: documentation to avoid malpractice. International Journal of Health Care Quality Assurance 18(2):123–129, 2005.
3. Acute Care Section of the American Physical Therapy Association: Common Terminology. Accessed at http://www.acutept.org/commonterm.pdf on March 9, 2007.
4. The Joint Commission: Official "Do Not Use" List. Accessed at http://www.jointcommission.org/NR/rdonlyres/2329F8F5-6EC5-4E21-B932-54B2B7D53F00/0/06_dnu_list.pdf

Using Abbreviations

Translate each phrase or sentence written with abbreviations into a full English phrase or sentence. Translate each sentence or phrase written in English into a sentence or phrase written with abbreviations.

1. Physician's orders:
to PT per w/c
turn Pt. qh

Translation:

_____

_____

_____

2. In medical record:
Dx: RA; R/O SLE

Translation:

_____

_____

_____

3. In PT note:
Intervention plan: See Pt. once per day, activities of daily living training including transfer training, correcting for balance issues as needed, ultrasound at 1.0 to 1.5 watts per centimeter squared to anterior superior aspect of right knee for 5 minutes.

Translation:

_____

_____

_____

_____

4. In OT or PT note:
c/o SOB p̄ bilat. UE PNF exercises.

Translation:

_____

_____

_____

_____

5. In medical record:
Dx: Multiple sclerosis ; R/O OBS

Translation:

_____

_____

_____

6. In PT note:
The patient has a below-the-knee amputation. Has used a patellar tendon bearing prosthesis with a solid ankle cushion heel foot for the past 20 years.

Translation:

_____

_____

_____

7. In OT note:
The patient's heart rate increased 20 beats per minute after only 2 minutes of self-care activities of daily living.

Translation:

_____

_____

_____

8. <u>In PT note:</u>
The patient ambulated in the parallel bars, full weight bearing left lower extremity, for approximately 20 feet twice with minimal assistance of one person for balance.

<u>Translation:</u>

_____

_____

_____

9. <u>In OT or PT note:</u>
Upper extremity strength is 5/5 throughout bilaterally.

<u>Translation:</u>

_____

_____

10. <u>In PT or OT note:</u>
Anticipated Goal: decrease dependence in transfers wheelchair to bed to moderate assistance within 1 week.

<u>Translation:</u>

_____

_____

Answers to "Using Abbreviations: Worksheet 1" are included in Appendix A.

Using Abbreviations

Translate each phrase or sentence written with abbreviations into a full English phrase or sentence. Translate each sentence or phrase written in English into a sentence or phrase written with abbreviations.

1. From Pt. care note:
Pt. c/o Ⓡ hip
pain p̄ amb ≈ 300 ft. + 1 c̄ a walker
FWB Ⓡ LE c̄ min. assist.
of 1 for balance.

Translation:
_____
_____
_____

2. You must write in the following:
The patient may be 50 percent
partial weight bearing left lower
extremity per verbal order of
Dr. Smith.

Translation:
_____
_____
_____
_____

3. Order written in the medical record:
D/C US in area of Ⓡ SI joint.

Translation:
_____
_____
_____
_____

4. Medical Dx:
Fx Ⓛ clavicle & subluxation
Ⓛ SC joint.

Translation:
_____
_____
_____
_____
_____

5. In physician's note:
FBS upon adm was over 300.

Translation:
_____
_____
_____

6. In physician's note:
Dx: Chronic renal failure.

Translation:
_____
_____

7. You must write in the following:
Manual muscle test reveals strength
4/5 throughout the upper extremities
bilaterally.

Translation:
_____
_____
_____
_____

8. <u>From the medical record:</u>
X-ray examination reveals fracture
of the left third metacarpal
immediately proximal to the
metacarpophalangeal joint.

<u>Translation:</u>

_____

_____

_____

_____

9. <u>Order for you to write:</u>
To occupational therapy for
activities of daily living per
verbal order of Dr. Jones.

<u>Translation:</u>

_____

_____

10. <u>In the physician's note:</u>
Imp: peripheral neuropathy;
R/O CNS dysfunction.

<u>Translation:</u>

_____

_____

_____

_____

_____

Answers to "Using Abbreviations: Worksheet 2" are provided in Appendix A.

II | Documenting the Examination

When a therapist sees a patient for the first time, the therapist performs an examination.[1] This examination leads to the therapist's evaluation and determination of the diagnosis, prognosis, and plan of care for the patient. Therefore, documenting the results of the examination performed by the therapist is a very important part of documenting patient care.

As mentioned in Chapter 1, the examination is documented differently in Patient/Client Management and SOAP Note formats. The SOAP Note organizes the information according to the source of the information. The Patient/Client Management Note organizes the information by the patient/client management processes that occur in patient care.

This section first presents the three subsections of the Examination part of the Patient/Client Management Note (Chapters 8-10). Then it presents the Problem, S, and O sections of the SOAP Note (Chapters 11-13). Worksheets follow the chapters to allow you to practice and gain confidence in documenting these sections of the two note formats.

It should be noted that the American Physical Therapy Association (APTA) is encouraging the use of note formats that more closely mirror practice, as described in *The Guide to Physical Therapist Practice*. The Patient/Client Management Note format closely aligns to the format encouraged by the APTA. Therapists who have been using the SOAP Note format for many years may have developed poor habits in documentation that are difficult to change. Therefore, a switch to a different documentation format may be more easily accomplished than a change of the SOAP Note format to align more closely with *The Guide to Physical Therapist Practice*. This text is offering both formats so that young therapists can use a format that will more closely align with the patient/client management process described in *The Guide to Physical Therapist Practice*.

5 | The Patient/Client Management Note: Writing History

The first part of the Patient/Client Management Note is the Examination. The Examination section includes three subsections. The first subsection is titled *History*. The second subsection is titled *Systems Review*. The third subsection is titled *Tests and Measures.*[1] Information belongs under History if it includes the following:

- **Demographic information** about the patient known as identifying information: This information includes the patient's name, address, admission date, date of birth, sex, dominant hand, race, ethnicity, language, education level, advance directive preferences, referral source, and reasons for referral to therapy.
- The patient's **current conditions/chief complaints:** This includes the onset date of the problem, any incident that caused or contributed to the onset of the problem, prior history of similar problems, how the patient is caring for the problem, what makes the problem better and worse, and any other practitioner the patient is seeing for the problem.
- **Patient goals:** This includes the patient/client and sometimes family goals for therapy as told to the therapist by the patient/client or family/caretaker in cases where the patient cannot speak for him/herself.
- The patient's **prior level of function:** This describes the patient's level of function prior to the most recent onset of his current condition or complaints. If the patient has a chronic condition, this includes the level of function prior to the most recent onset or exacerbation of his/her symptoms.
- The patient's **social history:** The social history includes cultural and religious beliefs that might affect care, the person(s) with whom the patient lived prior to admission and will live after discharge, available social and physical supports available to the patient now and that will be available after discharge, and the availability of a caregiver.
- The patient's **employment status:** This includes whether the patient works full time or part time, inside or outside of the home; is retired; or is a student.
- A description of the patient's **living environment:** This includes the assistive devices and equipment the patient uses, the type of residence in which the patient lives, information about the environment, such as stairs or ramps available, and past use of community services. Community services can include day services or programs, home health services, homemaking services, hospice, Meals on Wheels, mental health services, respiratory therapy, or one of the rehabilitation therapies (physical therapy, occupational therapy, speech/language pathology).
- Information about the patient's **general health status:** This includes the patient's rating of his or her health and whether the patient has experienced any major life changes during the preceding year.
- Information about the patient's past and current **social/health habits:** This includes alcohol and tobacco use and exercise habits.
- Information about the patient's **family health history:** This is a general screening for a family history of heart disease, hypertension, stroke, diabetes, cancer, psychological conditions, arthritis, osteoporosis, and other conditions.
- Information about the **patient's medical/surgical history.**
- Information about the current **functional status/activity level** of the patient: This includes information on everything from bed mobility, transfers, gait, self-care, home management, and community and work activities that apply to the patient's current situation or condition.
- A current list of all of the **medications** the patient takes.
- The **growth and development** of the patient: This includes the developmental history and is most applicable to pediatric patients.
- **Other clinical tests** that the patient has experienced: This includes laboratory or radiology tests, and the dates and the findings of those tests.[1–3]

Although the therapist makes every attempt to perform a complete examination of the patient, not every category may be used with every patient. For example, the developmental category may not be applicable to an older adult with degenerative joint disease.

Use of the Term *Patient*

Much of the information in the History section of the note is obtained from the patient or the patient's family, friends, or caretakers. Therefore, many statements in the History part of the note may refer to the patient. It is unnecessary to refer to the source of information unless information from two sources conflicts despite the therapist's attempts to clarify discrepancies, or unless the information is clearly the patient's opinion or belief and not factual or documented medically.

> example
>
> **Functional Status/Activity Level:** Pt. states she performs all transfers indep. & safely. Pt.'s daughter states Pt. lives in assisted living situation because Pt. falls frequently & needs help c̄ transfers at times.
>
> **Current Condition:** Pt. states she believes the pain in her foot is caused by her back.

Abbreviations and Medical Terminology

Appropriate abbreviations and use of medical terminology are expected. Correct spelling is necessary for the therapist to be represented appropriately as a professional. The most concise (yet clear) wording should be used. Full sentences are not necessary if the idea is complete (this varies from facility to facility). If the information does not conflict, it is not necessary to identify the source of the information.

> **example**
>
> **Wordy:** The patient's daughter stated that she talked with her mother and that her mother will go to the daughter's home upon discharge from the hospital.
>
> **More Concise:** Pt. will go to daughter's home p̄ D/C.

Organization

Other health care professionals reading your note need to be able to find the information in your note. Therefore, the use of headings or subcategories is important. The headings used are the same as the types of information included in the History subsection of the note. To which of the two following examples would you rather refer if you were looking for particular information?

> **example**
>
> 1. Works full time inside of the home doing data entry. Lives in a house c̄ 4 stairs to enter. Pt. rates general health as fair. No railings on the stairs. Denies major life changes during past yr. Sidewalk between garage & house is uneven surface. Lives alone.
> 2. <u>Social History:</u> Lives alone. <u>Employment:</u> Works full time inside of home doing data entry. <u>Living Environment:</u> Lives in a house c̄ 4 stairs s̄ railings to enter. Sidewalk between garage & house is uneven surface. <u>General Health Status:</u> Rates general health as fair. Denies major life changes during past yr.

In the first example, getting a picture of the patient's home status, work status, and health status is difficult. The second example is much easier to read and understand.

Every initial note should include applicable information on the patient's demographic information, current conditions and chief complaints, goals, prior level of function, social history, employment or work status, living environment, general health status, social and health habits, family health history, medical/surgical history, current functional status and activity level, medications, and other clinical tests. Growth and development is an optional subcategory. The information under each subcategory should be as brief and concise as possible. The purpose of the information is not to add length to the note, but to provide necessary documentation of the patient's history.

Progress Notes

Progress note formats for the Patient/Client Management Note vary. In some facilities, the History subsection of a progress note is written using only the categories that need to be updated. Other facilities use the SOAP Note format to document patient progress. Each individual health care facility has policies regarding how to document updates to the information included in the History part of the note.

Discharge Summaries

In some health care facilities, the History section of the Discharge Summary is used as a summary of the patient's history, including progress or changes made in certain areas during the course of care. Some subsections under History remain unchanged (unless the information was corrected) from the initial note. Other subsections summarize the changes made while the patient received therapy.

> **example**
>
> From a single subheading of the History section of the note:
>
> **Current Conditions/Chief Complaint:** Pt. initially c/o low back pain of an intensity of 8 on a 0–10 scale. Pt. was pain free upon D/C from PT. Pt. stated she learned she had to do her exercises daily to remain pain free.

Other health care facilities omit the History section from the Discharge Summary.

S u m m a r y   a n d   O b j e c t i v e

The History is the first section of the Examination part of the Patient/Client Management Note. It should include subheadings with information regarding the patient's demographics, current conditions/chief complaints, goals, prior level of function, social history, employment or work situation, living environment, general health status, social and health habits, family history, medical/surgical history, current functional status and activity level, medications, and other clinical tests. The history should be written concisely and with the use of appropriate abbreviations and spelling.

The worksheets that follow will give you practice writing the History portion of the Patient/Client Management Note. After reviewing the material in this chapter, completing the following worksheets, and using the answer sheets to correct the worksheets, you will be able to write the History subsection of a Patient/Client Management Note.

R e f e r e n c e s

1. American Physical Therapy Association: Guide to Physical Therapist Practice, ed. 2, and CD-ROM. American Physical Therapy Association, Alexandria, VA, 2003.
2. Defensible Documentation for Patient/Client Management. Accessed at http://www.apta.org/AM/Template. cfm?Section=Documentation4&Template=/MembersOnly. cfm&ContentID=37776 on March 9, 2007.
3. American Physical Therapy Association: Guidelines: Physical Therapy Documentation Of Patient/Client Management. Accessed at http://www.apta.org/AM/Template. cfm?Section=Home&TEMPLATE=/CM/ContentDisplay. cfm&CONTENTID=31688 on March 9, 2007.

Writing History

> **PART I.** Mark the statements that should be placed in the *History* category by placing an *Hx* on the line before the statement.

1. _____ Pt. best learns through reading and demonstration.

2. _____ Communication abilities: unimpaired.

3. _____ Pt. is a 31 y.o. white male referred by Dr. Smith c̄ a medical dx of S/P fx Ⓡ femur 6 wks. ago.

4. _____ Integumentary system: skin color and integrity WNL.

5. _____ Prior Rx: PT in ED for training in gait c̄ crutches.

6. _____ Lives c̄ his wife & 2 children.

7. _____ Pt. is indep. in all transfer, ADL, & IADL activities.

8. _____ Balance is not impaired.

9. _____ Oriented ×3.

10. _____ Pt. works full time as a postal worker & has been on leave of absence for past 6 wks.

11. _____ Education needs: exercise program & recovery process from fx.

12. _____ Pt. referred for gait training s̄ assistive device.

13. _____ Denies major life changes during the past year.

14. _____ Rates general health as excellent.

15. _____ Gross locomotion NWB c̄ crutches is not impaired; has been NWB Ⓡ LE for 6 wks.

PART II. Below you will find the headings discussed for the *History* subsection of the note. Each is followed by five blanks (more than are needed for the exercise). Below these headings are twenty statements to be included in the note. Write the number of each in the blank following its appropriate heading. The statements you list following each heading should be in the order in which they would logically appear in a note (for instance, 1-5-3 might make more sense than if you were to order them 3-1-5). You may wish to write the note out on a separate piece of paper to assist yourself with this task.

A. Demographics: _____ , _____ , _____ , _____ , _____

B. Current Condition(s)/Chief Complaint(s): _____ , _____ , _____ , _____ , _____

C. Pt. Goals: _____ , _____ , _____ , _____ , _____

D. Prior Level of Function: _____ , _____ , _____ , _____ , _____

E. Social Hx: _____ , _____ , _____ , _____ , _____

F. Employment/Work: _____ , _____ , _____ , _____ , _____

G. Living Environment: _____ , _____ , _____ , _____ , _____

H. General Health Status: _____ , _____ , _____ , _____ , _____

I. Social/Health Habits: _____ , _____ , _____ , _____ , _____

J. Family Hx: _____ , _____ , _____ , _____ , _____

K. Medical/Surgical Hx: _____ , _____ , _____ , _____ , _____

L. Functional Status/Activity Level: _____ , _____ , _____ , _____ , _____

M. Medications: _____ , _____ , _____ , _____ , _____

N. Other Clinical Tests: _____ , _____ , _____ , _____ , _____

1. Perceives general health as good.

2. Pt. lap swims 1.5 hrs. 5×/wk.

3. c/o pain c̄ wt. bearing Ⓡ ankle.

4. X-rays were neg.

5. Referred by Dr. Jones.

6. Unable to play bass in church (stands for this activity).

7. Home has 1 step to enter & is on 1 level.

8. Walking at school is painful.

9. Cannot stand during bass lessons.

10. 13 y.o.

11. Wears an ankle wrap when swimming.

12. Medical dx of S/P sprain Ⓡ ankle 4 wks.

13. Rates pain as 4 on a 0–10 scale (0 = no pain).

14. Female

15. Has not received any Rx of this Ⓡ ankle sprain other than splinting.

16. Hx of 3 previous Ⓡ ankle sprains & 2 previous Ⓡ wrist sprains.

17. Caucasian

18. Pain is limiting Pt.'s recreational activities in middle school; unable to participate in after-school art activities due to pain level at end of day.

19. Pt. wants PT to help her to be able to amb. pain free s̄ splint Ⓡ LE.

20. Lives c̄ parents.

21. Pt. does not smoke or drink.

22. Pt. is Ⓡ handed.

23. Attends middle school.

24. School has 2 levels c̄ 2 flights of 10 steps between levels.

25. Currently takes 400 mg. of ibuprofen TID for pain.

26. Is on swim team at local YMCA.

27. Pt. fell on a step at home & "severely" twisted Ⓡ ankle medially on [date].

28. Plays bass in orchestra at school.

29. Grandparents had HCVD, father has Htn, sister dx c̄ connective tissue disease; family could not remember name of connective tissue disease.

30. Currently wearing splint on Ⓡ ankle.

31. Had no difficulties or pain with ambulation or standing activities prior to current injury.

> ▮ **PART III.** Rewrite the following History statements in a more clear, concise, and professional manner. Also, list the heading under which the statement should be placed.

1. The patient is an 83-year-old woman who is African-American and who is right-handed.

   a. <u>Heading:</u> _____

   b. <u>Corrected statement:</u> _____

   _____

2. The patient fell and hit her right arm and her head as she was standing up from her sofa.

   a. <u>Heading:</u> _____

   b. <u>Corrected statement:</u> _____

   _____

3. The patient's doctor told us that result of the x-ray examination of the right arm was negative.

   a. <u>Heading:</u> _____

   b. <u>Corrected statement:</u> _____

   _____

4. The patient lives in an apartment in an assisted living complex and meals, laundry services, and housekeeping services are provided, and she can get help with bathing as needed.

   a. <u>Heading:</u> _____

   b. <u>Corrected statement:</u> _____

   _____

5. The patient told us that health care is "unneeded and usually dangerous."

   a. <u>Heading:</u> _____

   b. <u>Corrected statement:</u> _____

   _____

> ■ **PART IV.** The following are the notes to yourself that you jotted down while reading the medical record and talking with a patient. The information is from an initial examination. (While jotting down notes for yourself, you did not consult Nursing Home XYZ's approved abbreviations list.)

Information from Reading the Medical Record

98 years old

female

family concerned and visits patient frequently

stopped walking during the past 2 weeks

refuses to walk now for nursing staff

referred by nursing with approval of house doctor, Dr. Frien

Caucasian

the patient has high blood pressure that is controlled by medication

no other medications

family history of high blood pressure

the patient does not smoke or drink

until a month ago, the patient had been very active in recreational activities, including arts and crafts, bingo, and social activities, with the recreational therapist

routine urinalysis was normal 1 wk. ago

Information from Part of the Examination of the Patient

says she has had arthritis in her knees for more than 50 years

says the arthritis is not the cause of her refusing to walk

has to go to the bathroom frequently to urinate

has used a wheelchair during the past 10 days to get around the nursing home

says she gets herself into her wheelchair without help

says she quit walking because she couldn't get to the bathroom in time when she stood up

says she keeps a towel in her wheelchair at the nursing home just in case she cannot control her bladder

has had some bladder control problems for about 5 years but they have become more severe in past few weeks

says she could not tell the doctor about her urinary problem because women are "not supposed to talk with men about those things"

says she doesn't know if it is possible to walk any more because her bladder control problem is so bad

says she has not told the nurses about it because the head nurse is male and she has beliefs about men and women talking about problems with urine

says she has not had any kind of treatment for her problem yet

says she has not walked in 10 days

says she wants to have this problem improved so that she can walk to the far wing of the nursing home to the recreational activities

says cannot push the wheelchair far enough to get to the recreational activities

Write this information into the History section of a note.

_____

_____

_____

_____

_____

_____

_____

_____

_____

_____

_____

_____

_____

_____

_____

_____

_____

_____

_____

_____

_____

_____

_____

_____

_____

_____

_____

_____

_____

_____

_____

_____

_____

_____

Answers to "Writing History: Worksheet 1" are provided in Appendix A.

Writing History

> **PART I.** In the following you will find the familiar headings used for the History part of the note. Each is followed by five blanks (more than are needed for the exercise). Below these headings are statements to be included in the note. Write the number of each in the blank following its appropriate heading. The statements you list after each heading should be in the order in which they would logically appear in a note (for instance, 1-5-3 may make more sense than if you were to order them 3-1-5). You may wish to write the note out on a separate piece of paper to assist yourself with this task.

A. Demographics: _____ , _____ , _____ , _____ , _____

B. Current Condition(s)/Chief Complaint(s): _____ , _____ , _____ , _____ , _____

C. Pt. Goals: _____ , _____ , _____ , _____ , _____

D. Prior Level of Function: _____ , _____ , _____ , _____ , _____

E. Social Hx: _____ , _____ , _____ , _____ , _____

F. Employment/Work: _____ , _____ , _____ , _____ , _____

G. Living Environment: _____ , _____ , _____ , _____ , _____

H. General Health Status: _____ , _____ , _____ , _____ , _____

I. Social/Health Habits: _____ , _____ , _____ , _____ , _____

J. Family Hx: _____ , _____ , _____ , _____ , _____

K. Medical/Surgical Hx: _____ , _____ , _____ , _____ , _____

L. Functional Status/Activity Level: _____ , _____ , _____ , _____ , _____

M. Medications: _____ , _____ , _____ , _____ , _____

N. Other Clinical Tests: _____ , _____ , _____ , _____ , _____

1. Medical dx is fx (L) hip c̄ ORIF [date].

2. Walked for fitness every day prior to fx.

3. No significant medical/surgical hx.

4. Pt. ambulated s̄ assistive device & was indep. in all ADLs prior to hip fx.

5. House has 2 steps to enter c̄ no hand railing.

6. Ambulance took Pt. home from the hospital because Pt. cannot navigate steps c̄ walker.

7. Pt. c/o pain (L) hip when standing NWB (L) LE c̄ walker.

8. Lives c̄ husband.

9. Pt.'s parents died of heart disease.

10. Currently daughter has hired a baby sitter until Pt. recovers fully.

11. Husband is 79 y.o.

12. Pt. is 75 y.o. Asian-American female.

13. X-rays 1 wk. ago revealed fx (L) femoral neck.

14. Pt. is taking pain medication.

15. Pt.'s brother died of cancer at age 43.

16. Husband is home all of the time & can assist Pt. c̄ transfers as needed.

17. States health is good.

18. Denies medication for anything other than pain.

19. Describes 15 ft. from Pt.'s bed to toilet.

20. Denies hx of smoking.

21. Pt. wants to be able to ambulate indep. around her house.

22. Pt. is retired but provides day care services for her daughter's children.

23. Husband's back hurts when he assists Pt. c̄ transfers.

24. Only prior adm. to hospital was at time of daughter's birth.

25. Lives in a house that is on 1 level c̄ carpeted floor surfaces throughout.

26. Pt. also volunteers at a literacy program on Sat. mornings.

27. Husband helps with light housework duties & cooking s̄ difficulty.

28. Hx of drinking ~1 glass of wine/wk.

29. States she cannot ambulate or transfer s̄ assistance.

30. Pt. wants to be able to transfer indep.

PART II. Mark the statements that should be placed in the History category by placing an *Hx* on the line before the statement.

1. _____ Will refer to OT to assist c̄ dressing.

2. _____ DTRs WNL throughout LEs except diminished Ⓡ KJ.

3. _____ Amb training, beginning standing B/S & progressing to walker.

4. _____ Pt. goal is to amb. indep. c̄ walker 140 ft. (3 within 2 wks.)

5. _____ Pt. c/o pain Ⓡ foot c̄ amb. PWB c̄ a walker.

6. _____ AROM Ⓛ knee 0–90°.

7. _____ C/o itching & pulling in scar Ⓛ wrist.

8. _____ Rolls supine→sidelying Ⓡ c̄ max assist. of 1.

9. _____ Pt. wants to go to daughter's house until she no longer needs the walker.

10. _____ Rx at B/S OD:

11. _____ Medical Hx: TIA in 2006, ASHD, CHF

12. _____ Dependent in transfers supine↔sit, sit↔stand, bed ↔B/S chair.

13. _____ Pt. lives alone in a 2-story house; 5 steps c̄ handrail to enter.

14. _____ Pt. will be given written & verbal instruction in a HEP prior to D/C.

15. _____ Recommend home health care PT p̄ D/C.

16. _____ Pt. speaks very little English; speaks Spanish fluently.

17. _____ Skin in area of scar Ⓛ wrist is very taut & adhered to scar tissue.

18. _____ PTA Pt. exercised regularly.

19. _____ Pt. is oriented ×3.

20. _____ Education needs: safety, exercise program, ADL, use of assistive devices/equipment, nature of condition, & the recovery process.

> **PART III.** In the following you will find information that belongs in the History part of the note. A blank line precedes each statement. Following these History statements are the headings used in the History section of the note. Write the letter of the appropriate heading in the blank preceding each statement.

1. _____ The patient attends ABC Middle School and is in seventh grade.

2. _____ The patient was playing volleyball and she jumped up in the air and landed on her right hip.

3. _____ The patient's mother has a history of breast cancer and a right mastectomy in 1997 with no evidence of recurrence of the cancer.

4. _____ The patient has never used any kind of walker or cane or other assistive device before.

5. _____ The patient is taking Demerol for pain.

6. _____ The patient is on the volleyball team at school and practices volleyball daily with the team.

7. _____ The patient is 13 years old.

8. _____ The house the patient lives in has three steps to enter the house with a handrail on the right side going up.

9. _____ The patient is right-handed.

10. _____ The patient has not experienced any major life changes during the past year.

11. _____ The patient has had no previous injuries or hospitalizations.

12. _____ The patient has a medical diagnosis of subcapital fracture right hip.

13. _____ The patient lives in a house with carpeted floor surfaces except for the kitchen.

14. _____ The x-ray examination shows a subcapital fracture in the right hip with a pin in place.

15. _____ The patient complains of "excruciating pain" in her right hip when she moves her right lower extremity at all.

16. _____ The patient's father has a history of hypertension that is controlled by medication.

17. _____ The patient's mother can assist the patient when she returns home.

18. _____ The patient and her mother rate the patient's general health as excellent.

19. _____ The patient is female.

20. _____ The patient says she does not have a history of alcohol or tobacco use.

21. _____ The patient's developmental history is within normal limits.

22. _____ The patient is Caucasian.

23. _____ The patient lives with her parents and an 11-year-old brother.

24. _____ There is a history of heart disease in the patient's maternal and paternal grandfathers.

25. _____ The patient was referred to physical therapy by Dr. Frume.

26. _____ The patient's mother does not work outside of the home.

27. _____ The patient's school has no steps.

28. _____ The laboratory test shows that the patient's hemoglobin value is 10.

29. _____ The patient has not been out of bed yet.

30. _____ The patient wants to return to home as soon as possible and then to school when she is safe and independent with ambulation.

A. <u>Demographics:</u>

B. <u>Current Condition(s)/Chief Complaint(s):</u>

C. <u>Pt. Goals:</u>

D. <u>Prior Level of Function:</u>

E. <u>Social Hx:</u>

F. <u>School:</u> (substituting for <u>Employment/Work:</u>)

G. <u>Living Environment:</u>

H. <u>General Health Status:</u>

I. <u>Social/Health Habits:</u>

J. <u>Family Hx:</u>

K. <u>Development:</u>

L. <u>Medical/Surgical Hx:</u>

M. <u>Functional Status/Activity Level:</u>

N. <u>Medications:</u>

O. <u>Other Clinical Tests:</u>

PART IV. Write the preceding information into the History section of a note. Remember to use abbreviations and brevity in writing the note.

_____

_____

_____

_____

_____

_____

_____

_____

_____

_____

_____

_____

_____

_____

_____

_____

_____

_____

_____

_____

_____

_____

_____

_____

_____

_____

_____

_____

_____

_____

_____

_____

Answers to "Writing History: Worksheet 2" are provided in Appendix A.

chapter

6 The Patient/Client Management Note: Writing the Systems Review

The *Systems Review* is the part of the Patient/Client Management Note that reports the results of a brief examination or screening of the cardiovascular/pulmonary, integumentary, musculoskeletal, and neuromuscular systems, and the patient's communication, affect, cognition, learning style, and education needs. This part of the note represents the first hands-on part of the examination. Except for the cardiovascular/pulmonary information, the information gathered in the Systems Review is reported as either *not impaired* or *impaired*. More specific descriptions and measurements are written in the Tests and Measures subsection of the Examination report.[1]

After the Systems Review is completed, the therapist determines whether physical therapy is appropriate for the patient or whether the patient should be referred to another health practitioner, such as the patient's physician, or both.[2] At times the Systems Review may not be completed because the therapist notes something from the patient's History and part of the Systems Review that indicates the patient needs to see another health care professional for care.

> example
>
> **Excerpts from the HISTORY and SYSTEMS Review sections of the Examination**
> **History:** <u>Current Condition:</u> Pt. c/o severe pain Ⓡ ankle & numbness & tingling in toes on Ⓡ. Pt. states was injured at a softball game the night before & was sent home c̄ ankle wrapped in elastic wrap. States twisted ankle laterally & heard a "pop" at time of injury. Has iced and elevated ankle since injury. Called physician and was told to see physical therapist. <u>Other tests:</u> Pt. has not had an x-ray of Ⓡ ankle.
>
> **Systems Review:** <u>Cardiovascular/Pulmonary:</u> Severe edema noted Ⓡ ankle. <u>Integumentary:</u> Skin is stretched tight & is shiny in area of edema Ⓡ ankle. Toes are cold & blue. Pt.'s physician contacted & Pt. referred to ED for further care.

Categorizing Information in the Systems Review

An item belongs under Systems Review if any of the following apply:

• It involves basic **Cardiovascular/Pulmonary** information, such as heart rate, respiratory rate, blood pressure, or edema. The Cardiovascular/ Pulmonary System is rated as *impaired* or *not impaired* as a whole system. Individual measurements of heart rate, blood pressure, respiratory rate, and a general description of edema are listed separately under this category.

> example
>
> **Cardiovascular/Pulmonary System:** impaired. BP 140/85. HR 90 bpm. RR 20 breaths/min. Edema: pitting edema noted bilat. ankles.

• It involves basic information on the **Integumentary System,** such as integumentary disruption, continuity of skin color, skin pliability, or texture. The Integumentary System as a whole is listed as *impaired* or *not impaired.* Specific measurements are not reported in this section of the note, although basic information is listed.

> example
>
> **Integumentary System:** impaired. Wound noted Ⓡ anterior leg. Skin discolored around area of wound. Skin thin & fragile bilat. LEs.

• It involves the basic information about the **Musculoskeletal System,** such as gross symmetry during standing, sitting, and activities, gross range of motion, and gross muscle strength. The patient's height and weight are also recorded with musculoskeletal information. Specific range of motion and muscle testing is not reported in this section of the note. Each subcategory of this section (gross symmetry, gross range of motion, gross muscle strength) is listed as *impaired* or *unimpaired.*

> example
>
> **Musculoskeletal System:** Gross symmetry: impaired in LEs in standing. Gross ROM: unimpaired bilat. LEs. Gross strength: impaired bilat. LEs, Ⓡ greater than Ⓛ. Height: 5 ft. 6 in. Weight: 140 lbs.

• It involves the **Neuromuscular System,** such as gait, locomotion (transfers, bed mobility), balance, and motor function (motor control, motor learning). Specific descriptions of these are not reported in this section of the note. Each individual subcategory (gait, locomotion, balance, motor function) under the Neuromuscular System is reported as *impaired* or *unimpaired*.

> example
>
> **Neuromuscular System:** Gait unimpaired. **Locomotion:** transfers impaired. **Balance:** unimpaired. **Motor function:** unimpaired.

- It involves the patient's **Communication Style or Abilities**, including whether the patient's communication is age-appropriate. Specific communication abilities are reported as *impaired* or *unimpaired*.

> example
>
> **Communication:** age appropriate & unimpaired.

- It involves the patient's **Affect,** such as the patient's emotional and behavioral responses. Specific affective abilities are reported as *impaired* or *unimpaired*.

> example
>
> **Affect:** emotional/behavioral responses unimpaired.

- It involves the patient's **Cognition,** such as whether the patient is oriented to person, place, and time (oriented ×3) or the patient's level of consciousness. Cognitive abilities are reported as *impaired* or *unimpaired*, with specifics mentioned as necessary.

> example
>
> **Cognition:** Level of consciousness unimpaired. Orientation to person unimpaired; orientation to place & time impaired.

- It involves any **Learning Barriers** that the patient may have, such as vision or hearing problems, inability to read, inability to understand what is read, language barriers (need for an interpreter), and any other learning barrier noted by the therapist. It should be noted that the use of glasses and hearing aids is listed in the *History* part of the note under Living Environment: Devices and Equipment. If the patient uses assistive devices that compensate for visual or hearing barriers, these barriers should only be noted if the assistive devices are not available, are not sufficient to compensate for the patient's learning barrier, or if the patient requires additional assistance of some kind.

> example
>
> **Learning Barriers:** Hearing: Pt. understands best when able to see therapist's lips along with use of hearing aid.

- It involves the patient's **Learning Style**. This includes reporting how the patient or client best learns (pictures, reading, listening, demonstration, other).

> example
>
> **Learning Style:** Pt. learns best when rationale for exercises is given before demonstration.

- It involves the patient's **Education Needs**. This includes reporting areas in which the patient needs more education or information, such as disease process, safety, use of devices or equipment, activities of daily living, exercise program, recovery and healing process, and other education needs noted by the therapist. These are reported as a listing of all of the areas in which the patient needs education.

> example
>
> **Education Needs:** disease process, home exercise program, use of the back in ADLs.

Abbreviations and Medical Terminology

Appropriate use of abbreviations and medical terminology is expected, as well as correct spelling. Clarity and conciseness are important.

Categories Used to Report the Systems Review

The categories used in the *Systems Review* part of the note are very consistent. They are the following:

- Cardiovascular/Pulmonary
- Integumentary
- Musculoskeletal
- Neuromuscular
- Communication
- Affect
- Cognition
- Learning Barriers
- Learning Style
- Education Needs

Information that is outside of the usual information in each of these categories can be written if it is outstanding and makes a difference in the therapist's decision to continue to examine a patient or to refer the patient elsewhere. In the example given previously, the therapist noted that the patient's toes were cold, although this was not a specific examination technique listed under the Integumentary System for Systems Review.

Writing Progress or Discharge Notes

Because the Systems Review is used for screening a patient for the appropriateness of therapy and the need to refer to other practitioners, this subsection of the note is generally not included in Progress or Discharge Notes. In some facilities, discharge notes might include a summary of the Systems Review or a rationale for referral to another health care provider.

Summary and Objective

The Systems Review Section of the Patient/Client Management Note is the section in which the therapist performs some very basic general examination/screening techniques. This information helps the therapist to plan the rest of the examination and to decide whether the patient has a problem that physical therapy can treat. The categories or headings used in the Systems Review subsection of the note are consistent. The information recorded under these categories or headings should be written in a clear and concise manner and should use appropriate medical terminology and abbreviations.

The following worksheets give practice at the skills needed to write the Systems Review section of the note. After reviewing this chapter, working with the worksheets, and using the answer sheets to correct the worksheets, you will be able to write the Systems Review section of the note.

References

1. American Physical Therapy Association: Guide to Physical Therapist Practice, ed. 2, and CD-ROM. American Physical Therapy Association, Alexandria, VA, 2003.
2. American Physical Therapy Association: Defensible Documentation for Patient/Client Management. Accessed at http://www.apta.org/AM/ Template.cfm?Section= Documentation4&Template=/MembersOnly. cfm&ContentID=37776 on March 9, 2007.

Writing the Systems Review

> **PART I.** Mark the statements that should be placed under the Systems Review section of the note by placing an *SR* on the line before the statement. Also mark the History items with an *Hx*.

1. _____ Heart rate is 82 bpm.

2. _____ Gait is impaired.

3. _____ Pt. lives c̄ her mother & her son & his wife.

4. _____ Pt. has dx of type I diabetes for 30 yrs.

5. _____ Oriented ×3.

6. _____ Pt. to be seen 2×/wk. in OP clinic.

7. _____ Gross AROM & PROM Ⓡ hip is impaired.

8. _____ Locomotion (transfers, bed mobility) is impaired.

9. _____ Pt. has Htn controlled by medication.

10. _____ Pt. best learns through demonstration, practice c̄ cues, & then referral to pictures as memory cues.

11. _____ Medical dx is s/p AK amputation Ⓡ LE.

12. _____ Son's wife is able to drive Pt. to PT.

13. _____ Pliability of skin around scar is impaired.

14. _____ Pt. will amb. indep. c̄ prosthetic Ⓡ LE s̄ assist. device p̄ 2 mo. of PT.

15. _____ No integumentary disruption noted; Ⓡ LE is healed.

16. _____ Communication is age-appropriate.

17. _____ Rx this date: teach Pt. home exercise program of stretching & strengthening to bilat. LEs & UEs.

18. _____ Pt. describes overall health as good.

19. _____ Education needs include use of prosthetic Ⓡ LE & assist. devices, safety, rehab. process, exercise program, ADLs.

20. _____ Balance standing: impaired.

> ■ **PART II.** Match each Systems Review statement with the appropriate heading. More than one statement may exist for each heading.

A. Cardiovascular/Pulmonary System

B. Integumentary System

C. Musculoskeletal System

D. Neuromuscular System

E. Communication

F. Affect

G. Cognition

H. Learning Barriers

I. Learning Style

J. Education Needs

1. _____ The patient requires a hearing aid to learn and communicate.

2. _____ The patient's height is 6 feet and 2 inches.

3. _____ The patient's gross muscle strength is impaired in the right upper extremity and is otherwise within normal limits.

4. _____ The patient's skin texture is thin and fragile.

5. _____ The patient's emotional and behavioral responses are impaired when the patient's breathing is more difficult.

6. _____ The patient's locomotion is impaired.

7. _____ The patient has multiple small tears in skin in the bilateral upper extremities.

8. _____ The patient's blood pressure is 130/83.

9. _____ The patient's heart rate is 92 beats per minute.

10. _____ The patient's balance is impaired.

11. _____ The patient's posture is impaired.

12. _____ The patient's gross active range of motion is impaired in the right upper extremity and otherwise is unimpaired.

13. _____ The patient weighs 180 pounds.

14. _____ The patient needs to learn about the disease process, the value of exercise, safety, and the use of adaptive equipment and assistive devices.

15. _____ The patient best learns from demonstration followed by reminders in the form of pictures.

16. _____ Inspection of the patient's skin color reveals multiple small hematomas noted below the skin.

17. _____ The patient's respiratory rate is 30 breaths per minute.

18. _____ The patient's communication is age-appropriate.

19. _____ The patient's gait is impaired.

20. _____ The patient is oriented to person and place but is confused as to the date.

> ■ **PART III.** Using the categories and statements in Part II and using appropriate abbreviations and brevity, write the information into the Systems Review section of a note.

_____

_____

_____

_____

_____

_____

_____

_____

_____

_____

_____

_____

_____

_____

_____

_____

_____

_____

_____

Answers to "Writing Systems Review: Worksheet 1" are provided in Appendix A.

Writing the Systems Review

> **PART I.** Mark each heading that belongs under the Systems Review section of the note by placing an *SR* on the line before the headings. Also mark the History headings with an *Hx*.

1. _____ Functional Status/Activity Level

2. _____ Neuromuscular System

3. _____ Demographic Information

4. _____ Learning Barriers

5. _____ General Health Status

6. _____ Cardiovascular/Pulmonary System

7. _____ Medical/Surgical History

8. _____ Integumentary System

9. _____ Medications

10. _____ Social/Health Habits

11. _____ Communication

12. _____ Patient Goals

13. _____ Cognition

14. _____ Social History

15. _____ Affect

16. _____ Family History

17. _____ Education Needs

18. _____ Other Clinical Tests

19. _____ Musculoskeletal System

20. _____ Current Conditions/Chief Complaint(s)

21. _____ Living Environment

22. _____ Learning Style

23. _____ Prior Level of Function

PART II. Write the appropriate Systems Review heading on the line before each statement below. As a reminder, Systems Review standard headings include Cardiovascular/Pulmonary System, Integumentary System, Musculoskeletal System, Neuromuscular System, Communication, Cognition, Affect, Learning Barriers, Learning Style, and Education Needs.

1. _____ Blood pressure is 125/85.

2. _____ Heart rate is 80 beats per minute.

3. _____ Gross strength is impaired in both lower extremities.

4. _____ Height is 6 feet, 2 inches.

5. _____ Weight is 190 pounds.

6. _____ No scar tissue noted on either foot.

7. _____ Skin integrity is impaired. Open area noted on plantar surface of right foot.

8. _____ Gait is impaired.

9. _____ Respiratory rate is 13 breaths per minute.

10. _____ Communication is unimpaired.

11. _____ Skin color is impaired. It is red in the area surrounding the wound.

12. _____ Gross symmetry is impaired in lower extremities.

13. _____ Skin texture is impaired in both feet. It is thin and fragile.

14. _____ Gross range of motion is impaired in both feet and ankles.

15. _____ Oriented to person, place, time is unimpaired.

16. _____ Needs education in the disease process, safety, wound care, exercise program, activities of daily living, use of assistive devices, general foot care.

17. _____ Balance is impaired.

18. _____ Learns best by demonstration by therapist accompanied by home exercise program that includes illustrations.

19. _____ Does not wear glasses and sight is impaired as a result of cataracts.

20. _____ Locomotion is unimpaired.

21. _____ Emotional and behavioral responses are unimpaired.

22. _____ Edema noted in right foot surrounding the wound on the plantar surface.

PART III. Using the categories and statements in Part II, and using appropriate abbreviations and brevity, write the information into the Systems Review section of a note.

_____
_____
_____
_____
_____
_____
_____
_____
_____
_____
_____
_____
_____
_____
_____
_____
_____
_____

Answers to "Writing Systems Review: Worksheet 2" are provided in Appendix A.

7 The Patient/Client Management Note: Documenting Tests and Measures

Tests and Measures is the section of the Patient/Client Management Note in which the results of tests and measures performed and the therapist's observations of the patient are recorded. Tests and measures are measurable or observable and contribute to the evaluation of the patient and determination of the diagnosis, prognosis, and plan of care. Good tests and measures are repeatable, valid, and reliable. When tests and measures are recorded, the therapist can compare them with tests and measures recorded in the past to determine the effectiveness of the therapeutic interventions. Tests and measures thus serve as comparative data as the patient's progress is monitored and reevaluated.[1,2]

Categorizing Items Into Tests and Measures

An item belongs in the Tests and Measures part of the Patient/Client Management Note only if it is the result of a test performed by the therapist or an observation made by the therapist.

> **example**
>
> **AROM:** WNL throughout UEs & LEs except 120° ⓡ shoulder flexion noted.

Each profession has common tests and measures used by the profession for certain diagnoses.

Abbreviations and Medical Terminology

Appropriate use of abbreviations and medical terminology is expected, as is correct spelling.

The following pages discuss some methods of recording tests and measures. Use them as a reference. Clarity and conciseness are important.

Categories

Information should be organized, easy to read, and easy to find. To organize the data from tests and measures better and make them easier to read, the data are listed under categories or headings. The headings or categories used depend on the patient's deficits and diagnosis.

Information about the patient can be organized by the *types of tests and measurements performed*. This type of organization is helpful when the patient has deficits in several parts of the body or some type of generalized problem. Examples of headings or categories used for this type of organization include the following:

- Ambulation
- Transfers
- Balance
- Range of motion (ROM)
- Strength
- Sensation

Headings or categories can also be based on *areas of the body and functional skills*. Use of this type of organization is found when many of the patient's deficits are located in one or two parts of the body. Examples of categories include the following:

- Ambulation
- Activities of daily living (ADLs)
- Independent activities of daily living (IADLs)
- Upper extremities (UEs)
- Lower extremities (LEs)
- Trunk

> **example**
>
> **Poorly Written**
> **Tests and Measures:** UE Strength 5/5 except triceps. Amb c̄ standard walker NWB ⓡ LE ~2 ft. × 1 c̄ mod. assist of 1. ⓛ LE: Strength 5/5 except for gluteal musculature. Vital signs 3 min. p̄ amb.: BP 125/80, HR 85, RR 14. 4/5 triceps strength noted bilat. Able to manage NWB status ⓡ LE indep. 3+/5 ⓛ gluteus maximus & gluteus medius strength noted. ⓡ musculature controlling knee & ankle not tested this date 2° long leg cast. Transfers sit↔stand c̄ min. assist. of 1. ⓡ LE strength at hip 5/5 except gluteal musculature. Vitals at rest: BP 125/82, HR: 80, RR: 13. Transfers w/c↔bed c̄ mod. assist of 1. Able to wiggle toes ⓡ LE; further testing

deferred 2° recent trimalleolar fx. Transfers supine↔sit c̄ min. assist. of 1. 3+/5 Ⓡ gluteus maximus & gluteus medius strength noted. Vital signs immed. p̄ amb.: BP 140/85, HR 120, RR 20. Transfers on/off toilet c mod. assist of 1.

Properly Written
Tests and Measures: Amb: c̄ standard walker NWB Ⓡ LE ~2 ft. × 1 c̄ mod. assist of 1 **Transfers**: sit↔stand & supine↔sit c̄ min. assist. of 1; w/c↔bed & on/off toilet c̄ mod. assist. of 1. **UEs**: Strength 5/5 except 4/5 triceps noted. Ⓛ **LE**: Strength: 5/5 except 3+/5 gluteus maximus & gluteus medius. Ⓡ **LE**: Strength at hip 5/5 except 3+/5 gluteus maximus & gluteus medius. Musculature controlling knee & ankle not tested this date 2° long leg cast. Able to wiggle toes; further testing deferred 2° recent trimalleolar fx. Able to manage NWB status indep. **Aerobic capacity & endurance**: Vitals at rest: BP 125/82, HR 80, RR 13; vital signs immed. p̄ amb.: BP 140/85, HR 120, RR 20; vital signs 3 min. p̄ amb.: BP 125/80, HR 85, RR 14.

The following are also examples of categories:

- Ambulation
- ADLs
- IADLs
- Ⓡ Extremities
- Ⓛ Extremities
- Trunk

Use of categories varies from one clinical facility to another. Certain facilities require therapists to categorize information on all patients in the same manner despite differences between patients in diagnoses and deficits. (For example, all notes in one facility might have the categories *gait, ADL, IADL, strength, ROM,* and *sensation.*) This may be done to compare data across similar cases. Other facilities give the therapists more freedom to categorize information in the manner they deem most efficient and organized. For the purposes of this workbook, you are expected to choose the most appropriate categories for each patient's specific diagnosis and deficits.

Within the *Tests and Measures* portion of a note, the categories can be arranged using a number of different methods. Some clinicians list the functional activities (gait, transfers, ADL) first because they believe that functional activities are the most important. Others believe that the impairments should be listed first because specific information on impairments is needed to understand the reasons for functional deficits. Most of the audiences for patient care notes (physicians, insurance reviewers, lawyers, utilization reviewers, and social workers) prefer listing the functional activities first, with the impairments listed after the functional deficits. For

the purposes of this workbook, you are expected to address functional activities and deficits before listing impairments.

Within any individual category in the *Tests and Measures* subsection of a note, the information is organized in the most logical order possible. Usually one joint at a time is described, and joints are addressed from proximal to distal. Information is otherwise grouped as efficiently as possible within this framework.

> example
> **Test and Measures**: <u>UEs</u>: AROM: WNL except for 80° Ⓡ shoulder flexion & 90° Ⓡ elbow flexion. <u>Strength</u> (gross muscle exam performed): 4–/5 throughout Ⓡ shoulder musculature, 4+/5 biceps, 4/5 triceps, 3/5 musculature controlling the wrist & fingers. <u>Sensation</u>: Intact throughout.

Methods of Recording Data From Tests and Measures

In many facilities, complete sentences are not necessary, but information should be clear enough to get the idea across.

> example
> **Unclear**: AROM: ankle in cast.
> **Clear**: AROM: Ⓛ ankle not tested 2° short leg cast Ⓛ LE.

At times, using a table format gets the information across in the most complete manner.

> example
> **Strength**: Comparison of strength of LEs is as follows:

Musculature	Ⓛ LE	Ⓡ LE
Hip	5/5 all musculature	5/5 all musculature
Quadriceps	3/5	5/5
Hamstrings	2/5	5/5
Ankle and foot	0/5 all musculature except 1/5 anterior tibialis	5/5 all musculature

Sometimes a standard ROM or muscle testing chart, flow sheet, or some other standardized table can be used (many therapy departments have these available for use). Instead of giving detailed information within the note, the therapist can refer to the flow sheet or table and attach a copy to the note.

example

Strength: LEs: See attached table; limited Ⓛ LE.

A table or flow sheet should always be dated and signed and include the patient's name and medical record number.

Common Mistakes in Recording Data From Tests and Measures

Some of the most common mistakes in recording data from tests and measures are the following:

- Failure to state the affected body part
- Failure to state measurable information
- Failure to state the type of whatever it is that is being measured or observed

example

Correct
- AROM, the type of ROM measured
- Shoulder *flexion*, the type of movement measured
- *Gait* deviations, the type of deviations observed
- *Sliding board w/c→mat* transfers, the type of transfers observed

Writing Progress Notes

In a progress note, not every category addressed in an initial note is included. Use only the information obtained while re-examining the patient during therapy sessions. However, keep in mind that any test and measure describing a functional deficit or impairment in the initial note should be re-examined and addressed in a progress note in the future.

If a patient's status is unchanged and the area addressed is extremely important, it is acceptable to address the area and state that it is unchanged. However, for the sake of the reader, the unchanged status should be briefly described.

example

Correct
Transfers: Supine→sit still requires mod assist of 1.

When stating that the patient's status is unchanged, it is important to make sure that all of the tests and measures available have been used. In the previous example, perhaps the amount of assistance needed by the patient is unchanged, but the patient is performing the transfer more quickly (2 minutes to perform the transfer versus 5 minutes).

example

Better
Transfers: Supine→sit still requires mod assist. of 1 but performance of transfer requires 2 min. on this date (vs. 5 min. initially required). Transfer is becoming more functional.

Data used for comparison purposes can also be included. In the previous example, without the comparative data, the fact that the performance of the transfer required 2 minutes would seem insignificant to the reader. The reader may not take the time to look at a previously written note to obtain the patient's former status, or the reader may not have the previous note available.

If possible, stating a benchmark for reasonable function is extremely important. In the example above, stating, "Functional transfers in the home require performance of the transfer in XX seconds," might be helpful. If there is no professional literature available as a benchmark, stating one's professional opinion can be helpful. For example: "It is this therapist's opinion that functional transfers in the home require performance the transfer in XX seconds."

Information addressed in progress notes should include areas addressed in the last set of anticipated goals written. For example, if a goal is set for the patient to be able to roll supine→sidelying independently within 1 week, the patient's rolling status should be addressed in the Tests and Measures subsection in the next progress note.

Writing Discharge Notes

The completeness of the Tests and Measures subsection of a discharge note varies greatly among practice settings. In some facilities, the discharge note is similar to a progress note and is an update of the patient's status since the last progress note was written. In other facilities, the discharge note is a more complete summary of the patient's condition upon discharge from the facility. In these facilities, the Tests and Measures subsection of the note may list all of the functional deficits noted in the initial note with the progress from the initial note to discharge listed. The same may be true for impairments listed in the initial note, depending on the progress made.

Types of notes can also vary depending on who will be reading the note. For example, a note that is forwarded to a nursing home or home health agency might be a complete summary of the patient's condition, whereas a note that will go to medical records storage when the patient is discontinued may simply update the patient's status since the last progress note was written. The home health therapist or nursing home therapist may receive only the discharge summary from an acute or rehabilitation facility, so a more complete note is needed. For the purposes of this workbook, the discharge note is considered a complete summary of the patient's status on discharge and course of therapy, and you are to address all tests and measures used during the course of the patient's care.

Summary and Objective

The Tests and Measures subsection of the note is a very important section. It should be included in every note, whether it is an initial, progress, or discharge note. The information should be organized under headings, should be written in a clear and concise manner, and should list the results of tests and measures performed by the therapist.

The following worksheets give practice of the skills needed to write the Tests and Measures subsection of a note. After reviewing this chapter, working through the following worksheets, and using the answer sheets to correct the worksheets, you should be able to write accurately the Tests and Measures subsection of a note.

References

1. American Physical Therapy Association: Guide to Physical Therapist Practice, ed. 2, and CD-ROM. American Physical Therapy Association, Alexandria, VA, 2003.
2. American Physical Therapy Association: Defensible Documentation for Patient/Client Management. Accessed at http://www.apta.org/AM/Template.cfm?Section=Documentation4&Template=/MembersOnly.cfm&ContentID=37776 on March 9, 2007.

Documenting Tests and Measures

> **PART I.** On the blank line to the left of each statement, mark the statements that should be placed in the Tests and Measures subsection by placing *TM* on the line before the statement. Also mark the History items with an *Hx* and the information that belongs in the Systems Review subsection of the note by writing *SR*.

1. _____ DTRs normal throughout LEs except ↑ (R) KJ noted.

2. _____ Pt. was in a car accident & Pt.'s car was hit broadside on the passenger side.

3. _____ Will refer Pt. to OT to assist c̄ dressing.

4. _____ Expected Outcome: Indep. walker amb 150 ft. ×2 FWB within 2 wks.

5. _____ Amb. training, beginning in parallel bars & progressing to a walker, emphasizing normal wt. distribution on LEs bilat.

6. _____ Strength testing inconsistent because Pt. does not follow commands to hold against resistance.

7. _____ Learning Barriers: none noted

8. _____ C/o inability to dress indep.

9. _____ Transfers: Supine↔sit c̄ min. assist of 1.

10. _____ X-ray: Osteoporosis throughout lumbar spine.

11. _____ ↑ PROM (L) knee to 0–90º within 2 wks.

12. _____ Cognition: Impaired; oriented to person only.

13. _____ Proprioception: ↓ throughout (R) UE.

14. _____ C/o pain throughout (L) UE c̄ passive movement of the wrist.

15. _____ AROM (R) shoulder flexion: ↑ to 0–90º p̄ Rx.

16. _____ Will be seen BID at B/S:

17. _____ Pt. will be given written & verbal instructions in walking program & home exercise program for (R) UE strengthening.

18. _____ Sensation: Absent to light touch & pinprick throughout (L) L5 distribution.

19. _____ Pt. will demonstrate proper knowledge of back care & ADL p̄ discussion of ADLs & IADLs c̄ therapist & through 90% correct performance on an obstacle course for back ADLs & IADLs.

20. _____ C/o itching in scar (L) wrist ~2 ×/hr.

> **PART II.** Match each Tests and Measures statement with the appropriate heading. More than one statement may exist for each heading. Place the answer on the first blank line to the left of each statement.

A. <u>Amb</u>

B. <u>ADLs</u>

C. <u>UEs</u>

D. <u>LEs</u>

E. <u>Trunk</u>

1. _____ LE AROM is WNL bilat except SLR bilat limited to 0–50°
_____ due to tight hamstrings.

2. _____ Transfers supine↔sit indep. but slow; requires 2 minutes to
_____ perform transfer.

3. _____ Spasm noted Ⓛ lower lumbar paraspinal musculature.
_____

4. _____ LE strength is WNL bilat except 3/5 Ⓛ plantar flexors.
_____

5. _____ Tenderness to palpation of paraspinals in L4–5, L5–S1 area.
_____

6. _____ Pain in back increased to 8 & centralized to L4–5, L5–S1 area
_____ c̄ prone extension exercises; Ⓛ LE pain 0 (0–10 scale used; 0 = no pain).

7. _____ UE AROMs & strengths WNL.
_____

8. _____ Trunk AROM is WNL; repeated flexion in standing & supine
_____ positions ↑ pain in low back & Ⓛ LE.

9. _____ Posture: ↓ lumbar lordosis, head held in forward position, ↑
_____ thoracic kyphosis.

10. _____ Amb indep. s̄ device indep. but slow c̄ little trunk rotation
_____ noted; amb. 30 ft. in 1 min.

11. _____ Ankle jerk ↓ on Ⓛ, normal on Ⓡ.
_____

12. _____ SLR: + at 45° Ⓛ, - on Ⓡ.
_____

13. _____ Demonstrates improper lifting techniques when asked to lift a
_____ box & when asked to transfer Pts.

14. _____ LE sensation to light touch & pinprick is diminished in
_____ Ⓡ L5 dermatome; otherwise WNL.

15. _____ Repeated trunk extension in standing ↓ pain.

> **PART III.** On the second blank to the left of each of the previous statements, mark whether the Tests and Measures statement discusses function (write Func on the line) or a physical impairment (write Impair on the line).

> **PART IV.** The following are the notes to yourself that you jotted down while performing the tests and measures part of your examination. (While taking notes for yourself, you did not consult Hospital XYZ's approved abbreviations list.)

1. sit↔stand minimal +1 assist

2. parallel bars—stood minimal +1 assist for 1 min. twice then took 1 step c̄ minimal +1—FWB both LEs

3. LE strength at least 3/5 (group muscle test)—unable to test further due to mental status

4. UE strength at least 3/5 (group muscle test)—unable to test further due to mental status

5. all ROM WNL except 90º shoulder abduction & 110 degrees shoulder flexion bilaterally

6. fatigued after standing twice, all other examination deferred—too fatigued

Place an "X" before the headings you would use to write the Tests and Measures portion of this note.

_____ UEs

_____ LEs

_____ trunk

_____ transfers

_____ ambulation

_____ activity tolerance

_____ strength

_____ AROM

_____ (R) extremities

_____ ADL

_____ (L) extremities

> **PART V.** Following, you will find headings for the Tests and Measures portion of the note. (These headings were chosen because they require the least repetition.) Each heading is followed by five blanks (more than are needed for the exercise). Using the statements in Part IV of this worksheet, write the number of each after its appropriate heading. The information you list after each heading should be in the order in which information would logically appear in a note (for instance, 1-5-3 may make more sense than if you were to order them 3-1-5).

A. Ambulation: _____, _____, _____, _____, _____

B. Transfers: _____, _____, _____, _____, _____

C. Activity tolerance: _____, _____, _____, _____, _____

D. Strength: _____, _____, _____, _____, _____

E. AROM: _____, _____, _____, _____, _____

PART VI. Using the categories listed in Part V, write the information into the Tests and Measures portion of a note. Your partial note should be written to be an acceptable part of the patient's medical record at Hospital XYZ (using approved abbreviations).

TESTS & MEASURES: _____

_____

_____

_____

_____

_____

Answers to Tests and Measures: Worksheet 1 are provided in Appendix A.

Documenting Tests and Measures

> ◼ **PART I.** In the following you will find familiar headings discussed for the Tests and Measures portion of a progress note. Each heading is followed by five blanks (more than are needed for the exercise). Below these headings are seven statements to be included in the note. Write the number of each after its appropriate heading. The statements you list after each heading should be in the order in which they would logically appear in a note (for instance, 1-5-3 may make more sense than if you were to order them 3-1-5). You may wish to write the note out on a separate piece of paper to assist you with this task.

A. Ambulation: _____, _____, _____, _____, _____

B. Transfers: _____, _____, _____, _____, _____

C. Strength: _____, _____, _____, _____, _____

1. Sit→stand c̄ min +1 assist. & verbal cues for hand placement.

2. Stand→sit c̄ mod +1 assist.; Pt. does not reach for chair ā attempting to sit.

3. Amb 100 ft ×3 c̄ walker & min +1 assist.

4. Sit→supine c̄ standby assist. of 1 & verbal cues.

5. Supine→sit c̄ mod assist. of 1.

6. Bilat LE strength 4–/5 throughout; gross muscle testing performed.

7. Has difficulty turning c̄ walker.

> **PART II.** The following is a note written by a student. Using the same information, rewrite this Tests and Measures portion of the note using different categories and more concise writing, if and when possible.

TESTS & MEASURES: <u>Appearance:</u> Incision Ⓡ anterior forearm covered c̄ steri-strips. <u>AROM:</u> Ⓡ UE limited shoulder flexion to approx. 120°, abduction to approx. 70°, full elbow flexion, –42° elbow extension, full wrist flexion, wrist extension to neutral c̄ full finger flexion. Ⓛ UE full AROM all movements. LEs full AROM all movements. <u>Strength</u> (gross break test used): Ⓡ UE shoulder flexion 3+, shoulder abduction 3+, elbow flexion & extension 4, wrist flexion/extension 4, finger flexion & extension 4. Ⓛ UE 5/5 all movements. Ⓛ LE 4 all movements. Ⓡ LE normal all movements. <u>Sensation:</u> To light touch & pinprick normal all 4 extremities. <u>Transfers:</u> w/c↔mat pivot transfer c̄ minimal assist. of 1, sit↔supine indep. <u>Ambulation:</u> c̄ walker c̄ minimal assist for 50 ft. once wt. bearing as tolerated all extremities.

TESTS & MEASURES: _____

_____

_____

_____

_____

_____

_____

_____

_____

_____

_____

_____

_____

_____

Answers to Writing Tests & Measures: Worksheet 2 are provided in Appendix A.

Writing the History, Systems Review, and Tests and Measures

Feb 09 25

> **■ PART I.** Indicate which of the following statements belong in the *History, Systems Review,* and *Tests and Measures* sections of the Patient/Client Management note. Mark them by placing an *Hx, SR* or *TM* on the blank line before the appropriate statement. (Some of the statements do not belong in the Examination part of the note.)

1. ~~SR~~ **TM** ___ Incision healing well, length 3 in. location immediately prox. to (L) thumbnail.

— 2. ~~Goal~~ ___ ↑ AROM (R) shoulder to WNL within 4 wks. c̄ 3×/wk. Rx.

— 3. _____ Will instruct Pt. in a home exercise program to improve posture & alignment (attached).

4. **Hx** ___ Pt's wife states he amb. indep. s̄ assist. device PTA.

5. **TM** ___ DTRs: 2+ throughout.

6. **Hx** ___ Medical dx: low back pain.

7. **Hx** ___ Pt. had past experience of PT for low back pain s̄ relief of pain.

8. **Hx** ___ C/o (R) LE pain in posterolateral aspects of (R) thigh down to the knee; pain intensity: 8 (0 = no pain, 10 = worst possible pain).

9. **TM** ___ Will attempt to perform manual muscle test on another date when Pt. is more rested.

10. **Hx** ___ X-ray: arthritic spurs L3–5 (R).

11. ~~SR~~ **TM** ___ HR 75 ā exercise, 95 immediately p̄ exercise, & 75 bpm 3 min. p̄ exercise.

12. **TM** ___ Amb s̄ assist. device indep. & s̄ deviations

13. **Hx** ___ Describes onset of pain immed. p̄ lifting a 50 lb. bag of dog food on 01/01/20XX.

14. _____ BID: hot pack to low back for 20 min.

15. _____ Pt's rehab. potential is guarded.

WNL = within normal limits

s̄ = without

PTA = prior to admission

BID = bidaily (2x/day)

> **PART II.** Rewrite the following History, Systems Review, and Tests and Measures statements in a more clear, concise, and professional manner. Also, list the subsection of the notes (History, Systems Review, or Tests and Measures) and the heading under which the statement should be placed. Remember, the date of the note should be listed prior to the word "HISTORY."

1. The patient complains of the left lateral knee pain that comes and goes.

   a. <u>Part of the note:</u> _____

   b. <u>Heading:</u> _____

   c. <u>Corrected statement:</u> _____

2. The patient doesn't have as much sensation in the left L5 dermatome.

   a. <u>Part of the note:</u> _____

   b. <u>Heading:</u> _____

   c. <u>Corrected statement:</u> _____

3. The patient states a doctor "looked in [his] right knee with a scope" on 02/02/2008.

   a. <u>Part of the note:</u> _____

   b. <u>Heading:</u> _____

   c. <u>Corrected statement:</u> _____

4. The patient says he had "surgery where they opened up my skull" in February 2008.

   a. <u>Part of the note:</u> _____

   b. <u>Heading:</u> _____

   c. <u>Corrected statement:</u> _____

5. Right leg passive range of motion is within normal limits throughout.

   a. <u>Part of the note:</u> _____

   b. <u>Heading:</u> _____

   c. <u>Corrected statement:</u> _____

> **PART III.** Here are the notes to yourself that you jotted down while reading the chart and examining your patient. (While taking notes for yourself, you did not consult Hospital XYZ's approved abbreviations, list.)

FROM THE CHART

Diagnosis is fractured right femoral neck on 01/12/2008.
A right hip prosthesis was inserted on 01/13/2008.
Patient is 65 years old.
The patient is male.
Physician is Dr. Sosome.
Hgb was 11 this morning.
You are seeing the patient on 01/15/2008.
You tried to see the patient on 01/14/2008 but patient was dizzy lying in bed and Hgb was 7.
Patient received blood transfusion on 01/14/2008.

From the Patient

Pain Ⓡ hip while standing 8/10, while lying (before ambulation) 4/10
No PT or OT before—no walker or cane before this admission—no tub chair or portable commode currently available at home—no other assistive devices used for dressing, bathing, ambulating
Fell at home and hit Ⓡ hip on side of bathtub
Lives alone—senior apartment building—elevator—curbs only
Apartment bathroom has a bathtub with a shower and shower curtain
Retired this year—was a teacher—still volunteers at elementary school 3 days per week, reading with small children
For recreation, patient watches her grandchildren and plays cards with friends. Watches toddler-aged grandchildren once per week and plays cards with friends 2 nights per week.
Would like to return to her apartment after discharge
(For PTs:) Would like to eventually ambulate independently p̄ device once again
(For OTs:) Would like to able to manage grooming and dressing by herself; would "settle" for Meals on Wheels
Walks approximately 2 miles 3 times per week
Does not drink alcohol and does not smoke
Describes herself as healthy.
Did not take medication prior to admission.

Systems Review

Blood pressure was 140/80
Initially pulse rate was 80
Respiratory rate was 12
gait impaired, locomotion impaired, balance impaired in standing and during ambulation, motor function unimpaired
impaired skin at surgery site; otherwise WNL
gross strength impaired on the right as is the range of motion
Communication is unimpaired
the patient's emotional/behavioral responses are unimpaired
oriented to person, place and time, unimpaired
patient wears glasses and cannot read without them—therefore, will need them for the home exercise program
likes to be shown by the therapist and then tries to imitate therapist's actions—visual learner
needs to learn how to use a walker on level surfaces and on curbs, needs to learn transfers, needs to learn to check for proper healing of wound, needs a home exercise program

PT Examination Performed

UEs—ROMs WNL except –5 degrees of right elbow extension
UEs—strength 4+/5 throughout (group muscle test)
ROMs in left leg WNL
Right LE—ROMs limited secondary to post-op restrictions to 90° hip flexion, full active hip abduction, 0° hip medial and lateral rotation, 0° adduction
Left LE—strength 4+/5 throughout (group muscle tests)
Right LE—strength at least 3/5 throughout—not further examined due to recent surgery
w/c to and from bed transfer with moderate of 1 person
Sit to and from stand with minimal of 1 person
Supine to and from sit with moderate of 1 person
Ambulated—parallel bars minimal of 1 approximately 20 feet once 50% PWB right LE—felt dizzy and nauseated—no further examination or interventions performed this date—nurses notified
BP 145/90 immediately after ambulation, 135/80 3 min. after ambulation
Pulse 105 immediately after ambulation, 82 3 min. after ambulation
Breathing rate 18 immediately after ambulation; 12 3 minutes after ambulation

OT Examination Performed

UE strength 4+/5 throughout (group muscle test)
UE—AROM WNL except –5 degrees right elbow extension
Fine motor skills within normal limits
Transfers supine to and from sit with moderate assistance of 1
Transfers wheelchair to and from bed with moderate of 1
Patient initially seen bedside for assessment of grooming and dressing skills
Currently has IV infusing in left forearm
Patient able to bathe UE and trunk with supervison but needs minimal assistance of 1 for both LEs and needs setup for sponge bath
Able to groom his hair independently
Able to care for his teeth independently
Wears contact lenses; able to care for lenses by himself from a wheelchair
Dressing not assessed this date due to high pain level and low patient endurance

Write the preceding information into the History, Systems Review, and Tests and Measures portions of either a physical therapy note or an occupational therapy note. Your partial note should be written to be an acceptable part of the patient's medical record at Hospital XYZ. Remember to include a date prior to the History section of the note.

_____
_____
_____
_____
_____
_____
_____
_____
_____
_____
_____
_____
_____
_____
_____
_____
_____
_____
_____
_____
_____
_____
_____
_____
_____
_____
_____
_____
_____
_____
_____
_____
_____
_____
_____
_____

Answers to Review Worksheet: History, Systems Review, and Tests and Measures can be found in Appendix A.

8 The SOAP Note: Stating the Problem

*T*he *Problem* or *Diagnosis* is the first section of the SOAP Note. While learning how to write in the SOAP note format, you will notice you are using the same information that you used to write in the Patient/Client Management Note format, but you are organizing according to the source of the information instead of the type of information. It is important to be sure that the information that you are documenting in SOAP Note format represents best practice.[1] If it does not, the Patient/Client Management Note format would be more desirable.

In many facilities, the major problem or problems that have brought the patient to you for treatment are stated before actually beginning the SOAP note itself. This is usually stated as *Problem* or *Dx*. The Problem part of the note can be stated as the patient's chief complaint, the diagnosis, or a loss of function. It may be medical, psychological, or functional.

In some facilities the pertinent history or medical information taken from the chart is included in the Problem area. In others it is the first information written in the Objective part of the note. For the purposes of this workbook, you are expected to state this information in the Problem area of the note, because it is not the result of tests you have conducted (your interview or measurements). Information that follows may be included in the Problem part of a SOAP Note.

- **Demographic information** about the patient known as identifying information: This information includes the patient's name, address, admission date, date of birth, sex, dominant hand, race, ethnicity, language, education level, advance directive preferences, referral source, and reasons for referral to therapy.
- **Recent or past surgeries** affecting the present condition or treatment (e.g., hx of Ⓡ total knee replacement performed on [date]).
- **Past medical history** affecting the present condition or treatment (e.g., hx of CVA in March of 2008).
- **Present conditions/diseases** affecting the present condition or treatment (e.g., hypertension, CHF).
- **Medical test results** affecting the present condition or treatment (e.g., x-ray reveals fx Ⓛ tibial plateau).
- **Patient medications** if your source of information regarding patient medications is from the medical record and not the patient.

Examples of the Problem part of the note are as follows:

> **example**
>
> 1. Medical Dx: Ⓛ hemiplegia resulting from craniotomy for removal of tumor on 09-12-20XX. Hx of Htn. Referring physician: Dr. Alexad.
> 2. Problem: 58-yr.-old ♂ c̄ Ⓛ BK amputation on 02-17-2008 2° PVD. Hx of diabetes. Referring physician: Dr. Ollandern.

There are no worksheets on writing the problem. As you practice writing notes on the worksheets that follow, you are expected to state the problem (if it is given to you) before you write the rest of the note. You will get much practice at stating the problem in completing this workbook.

Reference

1. American Physical Therapy Association: Defensible Documentation for Patient/Client Management. Accessed at http://www.apta.org/AM/ Template.cfm?Section= Documentation4&Template=/MembersOnly. cfm&ContentID=37776 on March 9, 2007.

9 The SOAP Note: Writing Subjective (S)

The *Subjective (S)* part of the note is the section in which the therapist is able to state the information received from the patient or caretaker that is relevant to the patient's present condition. Subjective information is necessary to plan the objective assessment of the patient and to justify or explain certain goals that are set with the patient. For example, third-party payors, utilization review auditors, and quality assurance auditors may question testing a patient's ability to go up and down a flight of 16 steps or teaching a patient to go up and down those steps (and why it is taking the patient longer than other patients his age to become independent) unless the Subjective part of the note includes documentation that the patient has 16 steps to enter his home.

Categorizing Items as Subjective

An item belongs in the Subjective category if any of the following apply:

- *The patient* (or significant other) tells the therapist or assistant about the patient's **current conditions/chief complaints.** This includes the onset date of the problem, any incident that caused or contributed to the onset of the problem, prior history of similar problems, how the patient is caring for the problem, what makes the problem better and worse, and any other health care provider the patient is seeing for the problem. After the initial examination, the patient may report how a level of pain or his/her level of function has changed after receiving therapy.

- The *patient* or significant other/caretaker tells the therapist about his/her **prior level of function.** This describes the patient's level of function prior to the most recent onset of his current condition or complaints. If the patient has a chronic condition, this includes the level of function prior to the most recent onset or exacerbation of his/her symptoms.

- *The patient* tells the therapist the **patient's goals** for therapy. In instances in which the patient cannot speak for him/herself, the family or caretaker may become involved in setting goals for therapy.

- *The patient* (or significant other) tells the therapist or assistant about his or her cultural and religious beliefs that might affect care, the person(s) with whom the patient lived prior to admission and will live with at discharge, available social and physical supports the patient has now and will have at discharge, and the availability of a caregiver. This is referred to as **social history.**

- *The patient* (or significant other) tells the therapist or assistant whether he or she works full time or part time, inside or outside of the home; is retired; or is a student. This is referred to as **employment status.**

- *The patient* (or significant other) tells the therapist or assistant the assistive devices and equipment the patient uses; the type of residence in which the patient lives; information about the living environment such as stairs or ramps available; and past use of community services, including day services and programs, home health services, homemaking services, hospice, Meals on Wheels, mental health services, respiratory therapy, or rehabilitation therapy (physical therapy, occupational therapy, speech-language pathology). This is referred to as **living environment.**

- *The patient* (or significant other) tells the therapist or assistant about the patient's **general health status.** This includes a rating of the patient's health and whether the patient has experienced any major life changes during the past year.

- *The patient* (or significant other) tells the therapist or assistant about the patient's past and current **social/ health habits,** such as alcohol and tobacco use and exercise habits.

- *The patient* (or significant other) tells the therapist or assistant about the patient's **family health history.** This is a general screening for a family history of heart disease, hypertension, stroke, diabetes, cancer, psychological conditions, arthritis, osteoporosis, and other conditions.

- *The patient* (or significant other) tells the therapist or assistant about the activities that the patient can no longer perform as a result of the patient's current condition. This includes information on everything from bed mobility, transfers, ambulation, self-care, and home management, to community and work activities that apply to the patient's current situation or condition. This is often referred to as **functional status/ activity level** of the patient.

- *The patient* (or significant other) tells the therapist or assistant about the patient's **medical/surgical history.**

- *The patient* (or significant other) tells or gives the therapist or assistant a list of all of the **medications** the patient takes.

- *The patient* (or significant other) tells the therapist or assistant about the **growth and development** of the patient. This includes the developmental history of a patient and is most applicable to pediatric patients.
- *The patient* (or significant other) tells the therapist or assistant about **other clinical tests** applicable to the patient's current condition that the patient has experienced, such as laboratory tests or radiologic tests and the dates and findings of those tests.[1-3]
- *The patient* reports a **response to treatment interventions** (e.g., a decrease in pain intensity).
- **Anything** *the patient* (or a designated significant other) tells the therapist or assistant that is relevant and significant to the patient's case or present condition is recorded.

The relevant history and other relevant information regarding the patient that is obtained from the chart may be stated under the Problem section (in some facilities, it is stated under the O, Objective, section). It does not belong under the Subjective section because it is not something that the patient (or significant other) tells the therapist directly.

Use of the Term *Patient*

Generally, the *S* section of the note should be as brief (yet complete) as possible. It is acceptable to use "Pt." the first time, but do not repeat it with every sentence. It is assumed, unless otherwise stated, that the information in this section came from the patient.

> **example**
>
> **Incorrect:** Pt. c/o pain in (R) low back area. Pt. states pain ↓'s s̄ rest. Pt. states is unable to work or perform most ADLs because pt. cannot sit greater than 5 min. 2° pain.
>
> *This is a waste of time and space!*
>
> **Correct:** Pt. c/o pain in (R) low back area. States pain ↓'s c̄ rest; is unable to work or perform most ADLs because cannot sit greater than 5 min. 2° pain.

Abbreviations and Medical Terminology

Appropriate abbreviations and use of medical terminology are expected. Correct spelling is necessary for the therapist to be represented appropriately as a professional. The most concise (yet complete) wording should be used. Full sentences are not necessary if the idea is complete (this varies from facility to facility).

> **example**
>
> **Wordy:** The Pt. states pain began ~3 wks. ago Wed.
>
> **More concise:** Pt. states onset of pain on [date].

Organization

It is important for the sake of the other professionals reading the note to organize the note by topic. Often, subcategories, or headings, such as *current conditions/chief complaints, prior level of function, patient goals, social history, employment status, living environment, general health status, social/health habits, family health history, functional status/activity level, medical/surgical history, medications, growth and development, other clinical tests, response to treatment* are used. To which of the two examples in the following would you rather refer if you were looking for particular information?

> **example**
>
> 1. Pt. c/o pain (R) ankle when (R) ankle is in a dependent position. Lives alone & must prepare all meals. Pt.'s goal is to play basketball again. Denies previous use of crutches. Denies any other pain or dizziness. Describes 3 steps s̄ a handrail at entrance to his home. States hx of a fall at home & feeling his (R) ankle "pop." States played basketball 3x/wk. PTA.
> 2. <u>Current condition:</u> c/o pain (R) ankle when (R) ankle is in a dependent position. Denies any other pain or dizziness. States fell at home & felt his (R) ankle "pop." <u>Living environment:</u> Describes 3 steps s̄ a handrail at entrance to his home. Denies use of crutches PTA. <u>Social/health habits:</u> States played basketball 3x/wk. PTA. <u>Patient goals:</u> Pt.'s goal is to play basketball again.

In the first example, getting a clear picture of the patient's status is difficult. The second example is much easier to read.

Initial, progress, and discharge notes should all include information documented in the categories *Current Condition/Chief Complaint, Functional Status/Activity Level,* and *Patient Goals.* Initial notes should also include the other categories listed previously because that information is needed for clinical decision-making and discharge planning.

Do not include information or subcategories in the *S* section of the note just for the sake of inclusion. The purpose of information included in any part of the note is to address the patient's present condition and problems accurately and to assist in monitoring progress, revising the patient's program, and discontinuing therapy when necessary. Information that is not relevant to the patient's present condition, levels of function, or need for function at home should not be included. Irrelevant information wastes time, makes the note unnecessarily long, and may confuse all those who read the chart for purposes of case management, quality care assessment, discharge planning, utilization review, or reimbursement. For further information on reimbursement issues, see Appendix D.

Verbs

S statements frequently contain a verb that indicates that the statement is subjective and not taken from the chart. Verbs frequently used are *states, describes, denies, indicates, c/o.*

Quoting the Patient Verbatim

At times, quoting the patient verbatim is the most appropriate method of conveying subjective information. Some reasons for using direct quotes from the patient or a family member include the following:

- To illustrate **confusion** or **memory loss.** (Example: Pt. frequently states, "My mother will make everything all right. I want my mother." Pt. is 80 years old.) This can be used to illustrate why progress is slow or why therapy interventions may be inappropriate at this time.
- To illustrate **denial.** (Example: Pt.'s daughter states, "She won't need home health PT. Once I get her home, she'll get right up." The patient is dependent in ambulation & lives alone.) This can be used to assist with appropriate placement for the patient and to protect the patient from a potentially unsafe environment.
- To **describe pain.** (Example: Pt. describes pain as, "like a knife stabbing right through my Ⓡ thigh.")

Using Information Taken From a Family Member

Information taken from an interview with a patient's family member can be included in the following manner:

> **example**
>
> **Problem:** Ⓛ stroke c̄ Ⓡ hemiparesis & aphasia.
>
> **S:** (All of the following information was taken from Pt.'s daughter. Pt. is unable to verbalize 2° aphasia.) **Prior level of function:** Pt. amb indep PTA. **Living environment:** Pt. lives c̄ daughter & daughter's husband in a 1-story home c̄ 3 steps c̄ handrail Ⓛ ascending to enter the home. Home has carpeted & linoleum surfaces s̄ throw rugs. Pt.'s bedroom is ~7 ft. from the bathroom & ~15 ft. from the kitchen or living room. Daughter works full time. **Family goals:** Pt. must be able to stay alone during the day while daughter works.

Examples of using a combination of information taken from the patient and a family member follow in corresponding physical therapy and occupational therapy notes regarding the same patient:

> **example**
>
> **Problem:** Peripheral neuropathy bilat. LEs; COPD. **Medical Hx:** Htn, ASHD.
>
> **S: Current condition:** Pt. c/o SOB ā examination; immediately p̄ examination, indicated that SOB had ↓; 5 min. p̄ exercise, stated SOB had ↓. **Medical/surgical hx:** Pt.'s husband stated pt. hx of COPD for 10 yrs. & hx of Htn. controlled by medication. **Prior level of function:** Pt. has not amb for the past 2 mo. & has required assist. for transfers 2° SOB & weakness. Husband stated Pt. transferred & amb. s̄ assist. device indep. prior to past 2 mo. **Living environment:** Husband described a 1-story home; c̄ a ramp to access the entrance. All floor surfaces are linoleum. Farthest distance pt. must amb is ~50 ft. Husband is home full time to care for Pt. Pt. goals: Both stated long-term goal of Pt. amb indep, c̄ or s̄ assist. device, & short-term goal of indep. transfers.

> **example**
>
> **Problem:** Peripheral neuropathy bilat. LEs; COPD. **Medical Hx:** Htn, ASHD.
>
> **S: Current condition:** Pt. stated she cannot tolerate both PT & OT bid 2° fatigue. Husband states Pt. has needed assist. for dressing LEs, transfers w/c↔toilet & has required set-up for a sponge bath with assist. in bathing LEs. **Medical/surgical hx:** Pt. states 10 yr. hx of COPD. LE weakness began ~2 mo. ago. **Prior level of function:** Husband states Pt. was able to handle all self-care activities until 2 mo. ago. **Living environment:** Husband is home full time to care for Pt. but states he is having back pain p̄ transferring the Pt. **Pt. goals:** Both stated functional goal of indep transfers w/c↔toilet, indep in bathing & dressing, & Pt. would like to be able to bathe in the tub or shower.

Writing Progress Notes

The *S* portion of the note is optional in a progress note. It is used if there is an update of previous information or if there is relevant new information to convey. Listing information that reflects a temporary mood of discouragement in the patient is not necessary and could confuse those reading the note. Of course, irrelevant information is never appropriate.

Subjective information addressed in previously set goals for the patient should be addressed in the progress note. For example, the patient initially stated that his or her pain prevented the performance of functional activities and rated his or her level of pain using a pain scale. The therapist and patient set a goal for decreasing the patient's pain by three levels on the pain scale in one week. Because the pain level and functional activities were addressed in the initial examination and in the goals, the patient's functional level and level of pain should be addressed in the progress note at the end of the week. Although information such as pain level is subjective, it can be a method of showing progress when combined with functional progress.

A patient's subjective **response to treatment interventions,** such as pain following exercise, pain felt with movement, a decrease in pain after treatment, or fatigue after exercise, can be reported in a progress note. This information can be used to document improvement and reinforce objective measurements. For example, if a patient used to feel pain with exercise or a certain movement, such as bending forward or backward, and no longer feels pain, then the patient has improved in pain-free mobility, making him or her more functional in ADLs.

Another type of subjective information that can be addressed in the progress note is information regarding the **patient's compliance and/or other health conditions during the week.** After interviewing the patient, the therapist can document whether the patient is doing prescribed exercises at home and how often. (Example: Pt. states she is performing her exercises in th a.m. & late night time but performs exercises at midday ~50% of the time.) Medical problems, such as cold or flu, that could help explain why a patient did not progress during a week or two of therapy can be documented.

The patient's **functional status/activity level** is still another area that can be addressed in the *Subjective* section of the note. Unless the therapist sees the patient in the patient's home, she must rely on the patient to convey information about function at home. A patient may appear to be making only minimal progress in therapy on impairments of range of motion or strength (objective measures of the degree of impairment) but may be making large improvements in functional ability at home. Thus, subjective information regarding functional status should be included in progress notes.

Writing Discharge Notes

The completeness of the *S* section of a discharge note varies greatly from facility to facility. In some facilities, the discharge note is similar to a progress note and only updates the patient's status since the most recent progress note was written. In other facilities, the *S* portion of the discharge note more completely summarizes the patient's complaints, living environment, and functional status, comparing the patient's initial status to the discharge status. A discharge note may also list whether the patient believes the goals set were achieved and whether the patient feels ready to function at home. For the purposes of this workbook, the discharge note is to be considered a complete summary of the patient's status upon discharge from therapy, and all of the relevant subjective information regarding the patient should be addressed.

Summary and Objective

The *S* portion of the note should include relevant information that will assist the therapist with deciding which tests and measures are needed, setting goals for the patient, planning the treatment interventions, and deciding when to discontinue care. Irrelevant information should not be included, but care needs to be taken to address the patient's current condition, as well as the functional status and living environment, both at the present time and prior to the onset of the patient's current condition.

The worksheets that follow will give you practice in the skills needed to write the *S* portion of a note. Also included are some exercises in stating the problem. After reviewing Chapter 8, "Stating the Problem," and the material in this chapter; working with the following worksheets; and using the answer sheets to correct the worksheets, you should be able to easily write the problem and subjective portions of a note.

References

1. American Physical Therapy Association: Guide to Physical Therapist Practice, ed. 2, and CD-ROM. American Physical Therapy Association, Alexandria, VA, 2003.
2. Defensible Documentation for Patient/Client Management. Accessed at http://www.apta.org/AM/Template.cfm?Section=Documentation4&Template=/MembersOnly.cfm&ContentID=37776 on March 9, 2007.
3. American Physical Therapy Association: Guidelines: Physical Therapy Documentation of Patient/Client Management. Accessed at http://www.apta.org/AM/Template.cfm?Section=Home&TEMPLATE=/CM/ ContentDisplay.cfm&CONTENTID=31688 on March 9, 2007.

Writing Subjective (S): (Also Included: Stating the Problem)

> ■ **PART I.** Mark the statements that should be placed in the S category by placing an S on the line before the statement. Also mark the information that belongs in the Problem portion of the note by writing Prob. on the line before the statement.

1. _____ Pt. c/o pain Ⓛ wrist.

2. _____ Pt. will demonstrate a normal gait pattern 95% of the time within 3 wks.

3. _____ Flexion in lying reproduces Pt.'s worst Ⓡ LE pain.

4. _____ Pulsed US at 1.5–2.0 W/cm² to Ⓡ upper trapezius for 5 min.

5. _____ <u>Strength:</u> 5/5 throughout all extremities.

6. _____ States hx of COPD since 2007.

7. _____ Pt. has good rehab potential.

8. _____ Will be seen by OT 3×/wk. as an O.P.

9. _____ States onset of pain was in July 2007.

10. _____ <u>Hx</u> (from medical record): CA of the colon c̄ colostomy in 2007.

11. _____ <u>AROM:</u> WNL bilat LEs.

12. _____ Pt. has been referred to home health services for further PT & OT.

13. _____ ↑ AROM Ⓡ shoulder to WNL within 2 mo.

14. _____ Denies pain c̄ cough.

15. _____ Will initiate OT post-op per TKA pathway protocol.

16. _____ <u>Medical Hx</u> (from medical record): Htn, ASHD, CAD.

17. _____ Pt. was unable to communicate verbally & did not follow commands well; thus, only limited tests & measures performed.

18. _____ Indep in donning/doffing prosthesis within 1 wk.

19. _____ <u>Gait:</u> Independent c̄ crutches 10% PWB Ⓡ LE for 150 ft. ×2.

20. _____ C/o pain Ⓛ low back p̄ sitting for ~10 min.

21. _____ Will inquire if Pt. can be referred to speech-language pathologist.

22. _____ States his goal is to return to work ASAP.

> **PART II.**   The following is information regarding several patients' diagnoses and chief complaints. This information was taken from the chart or received from the physician's office. Write the information listed in each case into the Problem portion of a note.

1. The patient is an outpatient, and the patient's diagnosis received from the physician is "right shoulder bursitis."

   Correct statement: _____

   _____

   _____

   _____

2. The patient had a right-side stroke approximately 1 year ago with residual left hemiparesis. He now comes to you as an outpatient. The patient's present diagnosis from the physician is "left shoulder subluxation." The patient is a 75-year-old white male.

   Correct statement: _____

   _____

   _____

   _____

3. The patient is an inpatient with a diagnosis of respiratory failure. She has a history of chronic obstructive pulmonary disease and congestive heart failure. She also has a history of hypertension.

   Correct statement: _____

   _____

   _____

   _____

PART III. Below you will find the familiar headings discussed for the *S* portion of a note. Each is followed by five blanks (more than are needed for the exercise). Below these headings are statements to be included in the note. Write the number of each statement in the blank following its appropriate heading. The statements you list following each heading should be in the order in which they would logically appear in a note (for instance, 1–5–3 might make more sense than if you were to order them 3–1–5). You may wish to write the note out on a separate piece of paper to assist yourself with this task.

A. Current condition: _____, _____, _____, _____,

B. Prior level of function: _____, _____, _____, _____,

C. Pt. goals: _____, _____, _____, _____,

D. Social hx: _____, _____, _____, _____,

E. Employment status: _____, _____, _____, _____

F. Living environment: _____, _____, _____, _____

G. General health status: _____, _____, _____, _____

H. Social/health habits: _____, _____, _____, _____

I. Family health hx: _____, _____, _____, _____

J. Functional status/activity level: _____, _____, _____, _____,

K. Medical/surgical hx: _____, _____, _____, _____

L. Medications: _____, _____, _____, _____

1. Pt. c/o Ⓡ shoulder pain "all over the shoulder."

2. States fell at home & landed on a step on Ⓡ shoulder.

3. States lives c̄ husband at home.

4. Describes pain as constant c̄ intensity of 6 (0 = no pain, 10 = worst possible pain).

5. C/o difficulty lifting heavy cooking pots & closing zippers on the back of her clothing.

6. States pain ↓ c̄ rest & is at its worst while Pt. is at work.

7. States she wants to be able to close her zippers & cook s̄ assist. upon completion of therapy.

8. Denies previous shoulder pain/stiffness/inflammation.

9. States was able to fasten all clothing & was completely independent with all cooking activities and activities of daily living prior to her fall at home.

10. States is seeing PT to↓ Ⓡ shoulder pain & ↑ Ⓡ shoulder motion.

11. Rates overall health as good.

12. States had x-ray & MRI of Ⓡ shoulder c̄ WNL test results.

13. States hx of htn.

14. States family hx of htn.

15. States husband is currently helping her c̄ ADL tasks at home.

16. Pt. is retired.

17. Pt.'s husband is retired & available to help her at all times c̄ ADLs.

18. Pt. has hobby of gardening & is unable to work in the garden at this time 2° Ⓡ shoulder pain.

19. Pt.'s husband does not help Pt. in the garden.

20. States drives herself to therapy.

21. States 85 y.o. husband no longer drives.

22. States lives in a house in which the kitchen has many overhead cabinets.

23. Takes [medication] for htn.

24. States drinks 1 glass of red wine/evening c̄ dinner; does not smoke.

PART IV. Rewrite the following *S* statements in a more clear, concise, and professional manner. Also, list the heading under which the statement should be placed.

1. States she had a fall in her living room. (Question: What information from the patient would make this statement more informative and useful?)

a. Heading: _____

b. Corrected statement: _____

_____

c. Answer to question: _____

_____

_____

2. States pain began around 5:00 p.m. a wk. ago Wed.

a. Heading: _____

b. Corrected statement: _____

_____

3. States she is sore today in her Ⓡ foot. (Question: What information from the patient would make this statement more informative and useful?)

a. Heading: _____

b. Corrected statement: _____

_____

c. Answer to question: _____

_____

_____

4. States she lives in a house. States she has two steps to enter her home. States the steps have a handrail that is on the right when a person is going up the stairs.

a. Heading: _____

b. Corrected statement: _____

_____

5. States the pain goes from her right hand up her right forearm today. The pain is allowing her to type for only 5 minutes at a time.

a. Heading: _____

b. Corrected statement: _____

_____

PART V. The following are the notes to yourself that you jotted down while reading the chart and talking with two patients. The first information is from an initial examination; the second information is from a follow-up, progress, or re-examination. (While taking notes for yourself, you did not consult Hospital XYZ's approved abbreviations list.)

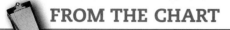

FROM THE CHART

58-yr.-old, male
Physician is Dr. Othrop
minor ligamentous injury ®️ knee
x-ray of right knee negative

From the Patient

®️ Knee pain—constant, "burning"—7 on 0–10 scale

↓ pain c̄ rest

↑ pain c̄ walking

No pain bending ®️ knee

Never used crutches before

Having difficulty walking

No prior difficulty with ambulation

Lives c̄ wife—apartment on 2nd floor—no elevator, 9 steps to enter c̄ handrail on the Ⓛ going ↑

Fell at work—landing on ®️ knee 1st

Wants to be able to access apartment independently (short term)

Wants to be able to resume former busy lifestyle, including returning to work as soon as possible (long term)

Occupation—carpenter

1. Write the previous information into the Problem and *S* portions of a note. Your partial note should be written to be an acceptable part of the patient's medical record at Hospital XYZ (using approved abbreviations).

_____

_____

_____

_____

_____

_____

_____

_____

_____

_____

_____

_____

_____

_____

_____

_____

FROM THE CHART

This is a progress note about an outpatient. You have received no new information from the patient's physician. For your information: the patient's diagnosis is minor ligamentous injury Ⓛ wrist. The patient is a 33-year-old male.

From the Patient

Ⓛ hand & wrist are puffy & feel stiff when the patient tries to move them

Puffiness worse after work

Types at work—up to 8 hrs. a day—MD told him to limit typing to 4 hrs. a day until stops swelling

Pain w/ typing—5 on a 0–10 scale

↓ pain w/ rest

↑ pain w/ grasping or wt. bearing activities Ⓛ UE

Having difficulty adjusting to splint—did not wear it due to rubbing on his thumb

Fell at work yesterday—landed on Ⓛ hand w/ wrist extended so pain has ↑ since last appointment

Went to physician yesterday—x-ray Ⓛ wrist and hand; told by physician that x-ray was negative

Wants to be able to hold a fork w/o pain (new short term)—trouble eating w/ Ⓡ hand—Ⓛ hand dominant

2. Write the previous information into the _S_ portion of the note. Your partial note should be written to be an acceptable part of the patient's medical record at Hospital XYZ (using approved abbreviations).

_____

_____

_____

_____

_____

_____

_____

_____

_____

_____

Answers to "Writing Subjective (S): Worksheet 1" are provided in Appendix A.

Writing Subjective (S): (Also Included: Stating the Problem)

> ■ **PART I.** In the following you will find the familiar headings discussed for the *S* portion of a note. Each is followed by five blanks (more than are needed for the exercise). Below these headings are statements to be included in the note. Write the number of each in the blank following its appropriate heading. The statements you list following each heading should be in the order in which they would logically appear in a note (for instance, 1–5–3 may make more sense than if you were to order them 3–1–5). You may wish to write the note out on a separate piece of paper to assist yourself with this task.

A. Current condition: _____, _____, _____, _____, _____

B. Prior level of function: _____, _____, _____, _____, _____

C. Pt. goals: _____, _____, _____, _____, _____, _____

D. Social hx: _____, _____, _____, _____, _____, _____

E. Employment status: _____, _____, _____, _____, _____

F. Living environment: _____, _____, _____, _____, _____

G. General health status: _____, _____, _____, _____, _____

H. Social/health habits: _____, _____, _____, _____, _____

I. Family health hx: _____, _____, _____, _____, _____

J. Functional status: _____, _____, _____, _____, _____

K. Medical/surgical hx: _____, _____, _____, _____, _____

L. Medications: _____, _____, _____, _____, _____

1. States fell at home & fx Ⓛ hip.

2. States needs to be able to amb c̄ walker indep. ~15 ft. to return home c̄ her husband.

3. States lives c̄ husband in her own home

4. Husband is home all day.

5. Describes 3 steps c̄ a handrail Ⓛ ascending at entrance of her home.

6. States hx of "bad heart trouble." but denies pain or difficulty presently. Cannot remember name of heart condition.

7. States used a walker since 1998 when she fx Ⓡ hip.

8. States is hard of hearing.

9. Pt. c/o pain Ⓛ hip c̄ standing NWB Ⓛ LE.

10. States would like to return home c̄ her husband p̄ D/C.

11. Pt. is retired.

12. Family health hx: Both parents died of MI p̄ the age of 80 y.o.

13. Currently feels she is in fair health.

14. Smokes 1 pack of cigarettes/wk; does not drink ETOH.

15. Takes [antihypertensive medications].

> **PART II.** Rewrite the following *S* statements in a more clear, concise, and professional manner. Also, list the heading under which the statement should be placed.

1. Pain is in her right leg down to, but not including, the knee. (Question: What other information regarding the patient's pain would help this statement to be more useful and informative?)

   a. Heading: _____

   b. Corrected statement: _____

   _____

   c. Answer to question: _____

   _____

   _____

2. States he depended on his wife to give him a bath before this stroke, and he plans to continue to depend on her to give him a bath now.

   a. Heading: _____

   b. Corrected statement: _____

   _____

3. Complains of not being able to put on her clothes by herself.

   a. Heading: _____

   b. Corrected statement: _____

4. Says she never used a walker before this present admission to Hospital XYZ.

   a. Heading: _____

   b. Corrected statement: _____

> **PART III.** Mark the statements that should be placed in the *S* category by placing an S on the line before the statement. Also mark the information that belongs in the Problem portion of the note by writing *Prob* on the line before the statement.

1. _____ Will request an order for OT to assist c̄ dressing.

2. _____ DTRs 2+ throughout LEs except 3+ Ⓡ KJ.

3. _____ Amb training, beginning parallel bars & progressing to a walker.

4. _____ States was in a car accident & Pt.'s car was hit broadside on the passenger side.

5. _____ Expected Outcome: Indep walker amb 150 ft. ×2 FWB within 2 wks.

6. _____ Examination not complete because Pt. does not follow commands consistently.

7. _____ C/o inability to zip her dresses behind her back.

8. _____ Transfers: Supine ↔ sit c̄ min. +1 assist.

9. _____ Proprioception: ↓ noted throughout entire Ⓡ UE.

10. _____ Medical hx: TIA in 2001, ASHD, CHF.

11. _____ C/o pain in "entire" Ⓛ LE c̄ active or passive movement of the knee.

12. _____ AROM Ⓛ knee to 0–90° within 2 wks.

13. _____ BID at B/S:

14. _____ Pt. will demonstrate knowledge of proper back care & ADL by discussion of ADL c̄ therapist & through 90% correct performance on an obstacle course in back care & ADL.

15. _____ C/o itching in scar Ⓛ wrist ~2×/hr.

16. _____ Will request an order for PT for assessment of gross motor functioning.

17. _____ Sensation: Absent to light touch & pin prick throughout L5 distribution on Ⓛ.

18. _____ Pt. will be given written & verbal instruction in home exercise & walking program (attached).

19. _____ States would like to return to his daughter's house until he no longer needs the walker.

> **PART IV.** The following are the notes to yourself that you jotted down while reading the chart and talking with your patient. (While taking notes for yourself, you did not consult Hospital XYZ's approved abbreviations list.)

FROM THE CHART

Diagnosis is contusion left hip.

Pt. is a 60 year old female patient of Dr. Grimee.

From the Patient

Ⓛ hip pain when FWB Ⓛ LE—8 on a 0–10 scale.

Total hip replacement Ⓛ 2000—used walker then.

No hip pain sitting or supine.

Apartment with elevator—curbs only.

Lives alone—husband died 10 years ago.

Fell in kitchen on Ⓛ hip in a.m.—able to get up s̄ help—pain throughout day—went to ED late p.m.

Did not use an assistive device before his injury and walked independently.

Did all ADL tasks independently prior to her injury.

Eventually would like to independently perform all ADL tasks s̄ walker.

Currently spends time in a wheelchair rented by the family.

Volunteers at her church—types church bulletin and helps clean.

Pt. is retired.

Pt. states she is in good health.

Does not smoke.

Does not drink alcoholic drinks.

Pt.'s mother has osteoporosis.

Pt.'s parents are living.

Write the previous information into the Problem and *S* portions of a note. Your partial note should be written to be an acceptable part of the patient's medical record at Hospital XYZ (using approved abbreviations).

_____

_____

_____

_____

_____

_____

_____

_____

_____

_____

_____

_____

_____

_____

_____

_____

_____

_____

_____

_____

_____

_____

_____

_____

_____

_____

Answers to "Writing Subjective (S): Worksheet 2" are provided in Appendix A.

chapter

10 | The SOAP Note: Writing Objective (O)

*T*he *Objective (O)* part of the note is the section in which the results of tests and measures performed and the therapist's objective observations of the patient are recorded. Objective data are the *measurable* or *observable* information used to formulate the plan of care. The testing procedures that produce objective data are *repeatable*. Objective information written in one note can be compared with the results of tests and measures taken and recorded in the past. It also serves as comparative data in the future, as the patient's progress is monitored and reevaluated. If objective data are not listed using repeatable tests and measures the SOAP Note format should not be used.

Categorizing Items Into Objective Notes

An item belongs under objective if the item is describing the **systems review** *done by the therapist.* The purpose of the systems review is to confirm that the patient is appropriate for therapy and to serve as a screening tool for referral to other health professionals. This is usually done during the initial examination of the patient.[1] The systems review includes the following:

- **Cardiovascular/Pulmonary System** information such as heart rate, respiratory rate, blood pressure, or edema. The Cardiovascular/Pulmonary system is rated as *impaired* or *not impaired* as a whole system, and individual measurements of heart rate, blood pressure, respiratory rate, and a general description of edema are listed.[1,2]

> example
>
> **Cardiovascular/Pulmonary System:** Impaired. BP 140/85. HR 90 bpm. Resp. Rate 20 breaths/min. Edema: pitting edema noted bilat. ankles.

- **Integumentary System** information such as integumentary disruption, continuity of skin color, skin pliability, or texture. The Integumentary System as a whole is listed as *impaired* or *not impaired.*[1,2]

> example
>
> **Integumentary System:** Impaired. Wound noted Ⓡ ant. leg. Skin discolored around area of wound. Skin thin & fragile bilat. LEs.

- **Musculoskeletal System** information such as gross symmetry during standing, sitting, and activities, gross range of motion, gross muscle strength. The patient's height and weight are also recorded with musculoskeletal information. Specific range of motion (ROM) and muscle testing is not reported as part of the systems review. Each subcategory of this section (gross symmetry, gross range of motion, gross muscle strength) is listed as *impaired* or *unimpaired.*[1,2]

> example
>
> **Musculoskeletal System:** Gross symmetry: impaired in LEs in standing. Gross ROM: unimpaired bilat. LEs. Gross Strength: impaired bilat. LEs, Ⓡ greater than Ⓛ

- **Neuromuscular System** information such as gait, locomotion (transfers, bed mobility), balance, and motor function (motor control, motor learning). Specific descriptions of these are not reported in this section of the note. Each individual subcategory (gait, locomotion, balance, motor function) under the Neuromuscular System is reported as *impaired* or *unimpaired.*[1,2]

> example
>
> **Neuromuscular System:** Gait unimpaired. Locomotion: transfers impaired. Balance: unimpaired. Motor function: unimpaired.

- **Communication Style or Abilities,** including whether the patient's communication is age-appropriate. Specific communication abilities are reported as *impaired* or *unimpaired.*[1,2]

> example
>
> **Communication:** Age-appropriate & unimpaired.

- Information regarding the patient's **Affect,** such as the patient's emotional and behavioral responses. Affective abilities are reported as *impaired* or *unimpaired.*[1,2]

> example
>
> **Affect:** Emotional/behavioral responses unimpaired.

- Information regarding the patient's **Cognition,** such as whether the patient is oriented to person, place, and time (oriented ×3), or the patient's level of consciousness. Cognitive abilities are reported as *impaired* or *unimpaired,* with specifics mentioned as necessary.[1,2]

example

Cognition: Level of consciousness unimpaired. Orientation to person unimpaired; orientation to place & time impaired.

- Information regarding **Learning Barriers** that the patient may have, such as vision or hearing problems, inability to read, inability to understand what is read, language barriers (needs an interpreter), and any other learning barrier noted by the therapist. [1,2]

example

Learning Barriers: Pt. is hard of hearing. Pt. understands best when able to see therapist's lips along with use of hearing aid.

- Information regarding the patient's **Learning Style.** This includes reporting *how the patient/client best learns* (e.g., pictures, reading, listening, demonstration, other). [1,2]

example

Learning Style: Pt. learns best when rationale for exercises is given before demonstration.

- Information regarding the patient's **Education Needs.** This includes reporting areas in which the patient needs more education or information, such as disease process, safety, use of devices and equipment, activities of daily living, exercise program, recovery and healing process, and other education needs noted by the therapist. These are reported as a listing of all of the areas in which the patient needs education. [1,2]

example

Education Needs: Disease process, home exercise program, use of the back in ADLs.

An item also belongs under Objective if either of the two following bulleted items apply:

- It is a **result of the therapist's objective tests and measures or observations** (must be measurable and reproducible data; may use database, flow sheets, or charts, to summarize data).

example

O: AROM: WNL throughout UEs & LEs except 120° Ⓛ shoulder flexion noted.

- It is part of the patient's **medical history** taken from the medical record and relevant to the current problem. Note: Only certain facilities include information from the medical record under the Objective section.

example

O: Medical Hx: ASHD, CHF, COPD. S/P fx Ⓛ hip c̄ prosthesis insertion 1 yr.

As mentioned previously, facilities differ widely as to whether information from the medical record becomes part of the therapy note, and if so, where and how much pertinent information is included. Some therapists believe that if the information is relevant enough to state, it should go with the diagnosis when the patient's problem is stated. Other facilities have a policy that information from the patient's medical record should be included in the Objective section of the note because it is information that the therapist did not obtain from the patient directly (and therefore is not subjective), and the section including the diagnosis is extremely brief. Still other facilities do not include information from the medical record under *O* because it is not a result of direct testing performed by the therapist. On arriving at a facility to practice, students should inquire as to which style of note writing is used. For the purposes of this workbook, you are expected to briefly include information from the medical record after the diagnosis or chief complaint when you initially state the patient's problem.

Abbreviations and Medical Terminology

Appropriate use of abbreviations and medical terminology is expected, as well as correct spelling. The following pages discuss some methods of recording objective data. Use them as a reference. Clarity and conciseness are important.

Organization

Information should be organized, easy to read, and easy to find. Please see the example in the next column.

Categories

To organize objective data better and make it easier to read, objective information is divided into categories or headings. The headings or categories used depend on the patient's deficits and diagnosis.

example

Poorly Written
O: Strength is 5/5 throughout UEs. ROM is WNL throughout UEs. Ⓡ toes are warm to touch & coloration is normal. Ⓛ LE AROM is WNL throughout. Ⓡ LE strength & ROM not assessed due to long leg cast. Ⓛ LE strength is 5/5 throughout. Able to manage NWB status Ⓡ LE indep.

Properly Written
O: TESTS & MEASURES: UEs & LEs: Strength & AROM are WNL throughout. Ⓡ LE: Strength & AROM not assessed due to long leg cast. Toes

warm to touch & coloration WNL. Able to manage NWB status indep.

A category or heading for the Systems Review should always begin the Objective section of a note. A heading for the results from Tests and Measures then follows.

Headings or categories in the tests and measures section of *O* can be based on the *types of tests and measurements performed*. This type of organization is helpful when the patient has deficits in several parts of the body or some type of generalized problem. Examples of categories include the following:

Ambulation
Transfers
Balance
ROM
Strength
Sensation

Headings or categories can also be based on *areas of the body and functional skills*. Use of this type of organization is found when many of the patient's deficits are located in one or two parts of the body. Examples of categories include the following:

Ambulation
ADL
UEs
LEs
Trunk

  Or

Ambulation
ADL
(R) Extremities
(L) Extremities
Trunk

Placement of Objective Data Into Subcategories

Placing objective data into subcategories depends on the diagnosis and deficits of the individual patient.

example

1. For the physical therapist, a patient with a low back problem may show deficits in the areas of gait, many aspects of the trunk, and the lower extremities, as well as body mechanics during transfers and activities of daily living. The information should be divided into subcategories that list the information regarding the trunk, lower extremities, and gait separately: *gait, ADL, trunk, LEs, UEs*. For the occupational therapist, the patient may show deficits in lifting abilities needed in her or his work, body

mechanics, and daily self-care activities. The information should be divided into subcategories listing the deficit areas separately: *vocational activities, body mechanics, self-care activities*.

2. A patient with a diagnosis of left-sided stroke might show deficits in many aspects regarding the right side of the body including decreased active movement, a change in tone, decreased sensation, changed deep tendon reflexes, decreased coordination, and decreased fine motor abilities. To make the information clearer and the deficits easier to read, the information regarding the right extremities should be separated from that for the left extremities because the left extremities are essentially normal. The trunk is one entity and should not be divided into different categories. Gait deviations and deficits in dressing and grooming exist and should each be described in a separate category. Deficits are found in other functional activities such as transfers and rolling. These functional activities can be listed under the subcategories of transfers and bed mobility. The subcategories used by the physical therapist might be *gait, transfers, bed mobility, (R) extremities, (L) extremities*, and *trunk*. The categories used by the occupational therapist might be *transfers, bed mobility, dressing, grooming, (R) extremities*, and *(L) extremities*.

3. A patient with colon cancer might show many deficits in strength and range of motion. These deficits occur in all of the extremities when the physical therapist assesses the patient. Transfers and ambulation need work. The patient's endurance is low. For the physical therapist, the information might best be divided according to the patient's basic areas of deficit: *ambulation, transfers, strength, AROMs, endurance*. When the occupational therapist assesses this patient, the patient also shows deficits in UE strength and AROM as well as deficits in endurance, feeding, grooming, and dressing activities. For the occupational therapist, the information might also best be divided according to areas of deficit: *feeding, grooming, dressing, UE strength, UE AROMs, endurance*.

4. When the therapist assesses a young pediatric patient, the assessment reveals low muscle tone, normal ROM, deficits in strength and stability, a delay in righting reactions, and deficits in mobility. These areas can all be listed under the category of gross motor skills. The child shows appropriate fine motor skills and deficient sensory functioning as well as difficulties in feeding. The therapist chooses to divide the categories into *ADL, gross motor, fine motor, sensory*.

Use of subcategories also varies from one clinical facility to another. Certain facilities require therapists to categorize information on all patients in the same manner despite differences in diagnoses and deficits among patients. (For example, all notes in one facility might have the categories *gait, ADL, strength, ROM, sensation.*) Other facilities give the therapists more freedom to categorize information in the manner they deem most efficient and organized. For the purposes of this workbook, you are expected to choose the most appropriate subcategories for each patient's specific diagnosis and deficits.

Within the objective portion of a note, the subcategories can be arranged using a number of different methods. Some clinicians list the functional activities (gait, transfers, ADL) first because they believe that functional activities are the most important. Others believe that the extremities and trunk or tests performed should be listed first because the information on specific impairments (ROM, strength, and so forth) is needed to understand the reasons for the deficits in function. Most of the audiences for patient care notes (physicians, insurance reviewers, lawyers, case managers, social workers) prefer listing the functional activities first, with the reasons for the deficits in function listed after the functional deficits. For the purposes of this workbook, you are expected to address functional activities before listing the impairments or specific tests performed.

Within any individual subcategory in the objective section of a note, the information is organized in the most logical order possible. Usually one joint at a time is described, and joints are addressed proximally to distally. Information is otherwise grouped as efficiently as possible within this framework.

> **example**
>
> **UEs:** AROM: WNL bilat. except for 80° ⓡ shoulder flexion & 90° ⓡ elbow flexion. Bilat. strength: 4−/5 throughout shoulder musculature, 4+/5 biceps, 4/5 triceps, 3/5 in musculature controlling the wrist & fingers. Sensation: Intact throughout bilat.

Methods of Recording Objective Data

In many facilities, complete sentences are not necessary, but information should be clear enough to get the idea across.

> **example**
>
> **Unclear**
> AROM: ⓛ ankle in cast.
>
> **Clear**
> AROM: ⓛ ankle not examined due to short leg cast ⓛ LE.

At times, using a table gets the information across in the most complete manner.

> **example**
>
> **Correct Method**
> **AROM:** finger & thumb extension/flexion is as follows:

Digit	MCP	PIP	DIP
1	20–0–45°	10–0–20°	
2	10–0–40°	0–15°	0–2°
3	10–0–40°	0–30°	10–0–5°
4	10–0–38°	0–10°	0–8°
5	20–0–47°	0–5°	0–5°

Sometimes, a standard ROM or muscle testing chart, flow sheet, or some other standardized table can be used (many therapy departments have these available for use). Instead of giving detailed information within the note, the therapist can refer to the flow sheet or chart and attach a copy to the note.

> **example**
>
> AROM 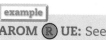 UE: See attached table; limited at shoulder & elbow.

A table or flow sheet should always be dated and signed.

Common Mistakes in Recording Objective Data

Some of the most common mistakes in recording objective data are the following:

1. Failure to state the *affected anatomy*
2. Failure to state objective information in *measurable terms*
3. Failure to state the *type* of whatever it is that is being measured or observed

> **example**
>
> **Correct**
> AROM, the type of ROM measured
> *Shoulder flexion*, the type of movement measured
> *Gait deviations*, the type of deviations observed
> *Sliding board w/c ↔ mat transfers*, the type of transfers observed

If a patient's condition cannot be stated in measurable terms, the word *appears* instead of *is* should be used.

> **example**
>
> **Correct**
> UE strength not formally tested on this date but appears functional for transfers w/c↔mat.

The term *appears* should be used very cautiously; third-party payors will not provide reimbursement for intervention that "appears" to be needed.

Some Specifics Regarding Recording Objective Data

Using scales with numerical values showing the value of normal, such as 3/5 strength, is suggested to make the job of those reading the notes for third-party payors somewhat easier. Appendix D includes some suggestions regarding recording objective data to maximize the effectiveness of note writing for third-party payors.

Methods for recording objective data along with common tests and measures can be found in *The Guide to Physical Therapist Practice*.[1]

Writing Progress Notes

In a progress note, not every category normally addressed in an initial note is included. Use only the information obtained while re-examining the patient during sessions subsequent to the initial examination and evaluation.[2,3]

If a patient's status is unchanged and the area addressed is extremely important, it is acceptable to address the area and describe briefly the unchanged status.

> **example**
>
> **Correct**
> **Transfers:** Supine ↔ sit still requires mod +1 assist.

When stating that the patient's status is unchanged, it is important to make sure that all of the tests and measures available have been used. In the previous example, perhaps the amount of assistance needed by the patient is unchanged, but the patient is performing the transfer more quickly (5 minutes to perform the transfer versus the 10 minutes the patient used to require).

> **example**
>
> **Correct**
> **Transfers:** Supine ↔ sit still requires mod +1 assist. but performance of transfer requires 5 min. on this date vs. 10 min. required on [date]. Transfer is becoming more functional.

Data used for comparison purposes can also be included. In the previous example, without the comparative data, the fact that the performance of the transfer required 5 minutes would seem insignificant to the reader. The reader may not take the time to look at a previously written note to obtain the patient's former status, or the previous note may not be available to the reader.

Information addressed in progress notes should include areas addressed in the last set of anticipated goals written. For example, if a goal is set for the patient to be able to "roll supine ↔ sidelying Ⓡ indep within 1 wk," the patient's rolling status should be addressed under *O* in the next progress note.

As mentioned previously, when writing notes, it is important to know the requirements of both the facility and the third-party payors. In most areas of the country, third-party payors require listing both the interventions the patient received and the patient's reaction to the interventions.[2] This can be listed in the *O* part of the note under **Reaction to Interventions**.

> **example**
>
> **Correct**
> **Reaction to Rx:** Pt. received 30 min. of gait training on this date emphasizing correction of gait deviations & correction of balance deficits. Responded well to verbal cues but could not cont. to correct gait deviations.

Writing Discharge Notes

The completeness of the *O* section of a discharge note varies greatly among practice settings. In some facilities, the discharge note is similar to a progress note and is an update of the patient's status since the last progress note was written. In other facilities, the discharge note is a more complete summary of the patient's condition upon discharge from the facility and, in format and length, is more similar to the initial note. Still other facilities use a format that summarizes the patient's condition upon beginning therapy, the general course of therapy, and the patient's status upon discharge from therapy.

Types of notes can also vary depending on who will be reading the note. For example, a note that is forwarded to a nursing home or home health agency might be a complete summary of the patient's condition, whereas a note that will go the medical records storage when the patient is discontinued may simply update the patient's status since the last progress note was written. The home health or nursing home therapist may receive only the discharge summary from an acute or rehabilitation facility, so a more complete note is needed. For the purposes of this workbook, the discharge note is considered a complete summary of the patient's status upon discharge and course of therapy, and you are to address all areas of objective data measured and remeasured during therapy.

S u m m a r y   a n d   O b j e c t i v e

The *O* section of the note is a very important section. It should be included in every type of note, whether it is an initial, progress, or discharge note. The information should be organized under headings, should be written in a clear and concise manner, and should list the results of observations, tests, and measures performed by the therapist. The first of the headings listed should always be the Systems Review in the initial note. The second heading should be the Tests and Measures in the initial note.

The following worksheets give practice at the skills needed to write the *O* part of a note. After reviewing this chapter, working with the following worksheets, and using the answer sheets to correct the worksheets, you should be able to write the Objective portion of a note easily.

R e f e r e n c e s

1. American Physical Therapy Association: Guide to Physical Therapist Practice, ed. 2, and CD-ROM. American Physical Therapy Association, Alexandria, VA, 2003.
2. American Physical Therapy Association: Defensible Documentation for Patient/Client Management. Accessed at http://www.apta.org/AM/Template.cfm?Section=Documentation4&Template=/MembersOnly.cfm&ContentID=37776 on March 9, 2007.
3. American Physical Therapy Association: Guidelines: Physical Therapy Documentation Of Patient/Client Management. Accessed at http://www.apta.org/AM/Template.cfm?Section=Home&TEMPLATE=/CM/ContentDisplay.cfm&CONTENTID=31688 on March 9, 2007.

Writing the Objective (O)

> **PART I.** Mark the statements that should be placed in the *O* category by placing an *O* on the line before the statement. Also mark the *S* items with an *S* and the information that belongs in the Problem portion of the note by writing *Prob.* on the line before the statement.

1. _____ Will receive pulsed US at 1.5–2.0 W/cm² to ®️ upper trapezius.

2. _____ <u>Strength:</u> 5/5 throughout all extremities.

3. _____ Pt. has good rehab. potential.

4. _____ Pt. c/o pain Ⓛ ankle.

5. _____ Hip clearing reproduces pain Ⓛ knee.

6. _____ States onset of pain in July 2005.

7. _____ Pt. has been referred to home health services for further Rx.

8. _____ Denies pain c̄ cough.

9. _____ <u>Dx:</u> traumatic brain injury.

10. _____ <u>Transfers:</u> w/c ↔ mat c̄ sliding board c̄ min + 1 assist.

11. _____ Indep in donning/doffing prosthesis within 1 wk.

12. _____ <u>Musculoskeletal System:</u> Strength impaired ®️ UE & LE.

13. _____ C/o pain Ⓛ low back p̄ sitting for ~10 min.

14. _____ Will refer Pt. to speech-language pathology.

15. _____ <u>Gait:</u> Indep c̄ crutches 10% PWB Ⓛ LE for 150 ft. ×2.

16. _____ Pt. was difficult to examine due to lack of cooperation as demonstrated by closing his eyes & crossing his arms when given a command.

17. _____ Will initiate OT post-op day 2 per critical pathway.

18. _____ ↑ AROM ®️ shoulder to WNL within 6 wks.

19. _____ <u>Reaction to Rx:</u> Received training in w/c propulsion & management, transfer training c̄ sliding board w/c↔mat & sit↔supine. Pt. was fatigued p̄ Rx.

20. _____ <u>AROM:</u> WNL bilat LEs.

21. _____ Will be seen by PT as an O.P. beginning c̄ 2×/wk. for 2 wks. & progressing prn.

22. _____ States hx of COPD since 2003.

23. _____ Pt. will be indep in dressing & grooming activities within 2 wks.

PART II. Match each *O* statement with the appropriate heading.

A. Systems Review

B. Tests and Measures:

1. _____ UE AROM is WNL except for 0–90° shoulder flexion bilat.

2. _____ ↓ sensation to light touch & pinprick noted in Ⓛ L5 distribution.

3. _____ LE AROM is WNL bilat.

4. _____ Cardiovascular/pulmonary: unimpaired. BP: 120/70. HR: 72. Respiratory Rate: 12. No edema noted.

5. _____ Amb pattern and speed is normal.

6. _____ All other UE sensation is WNL.

7. _____ Integumentary System: Unimpaired

8. _____ Strength is 5/5 in all extremities.

9. _____ Pt. was able to correct his gait pattern c̄ verbal cues p̄ Rx.

10. _____ Transfers supine ↔ sit are indep but too slow to be functional (5 min.).

11. _____ Pt. demonstrates ↓ time spent in stance phase on Ⓛ LE & ↓ step length Ⓡ LE.

12. _____ UE sensation is WNL bilat.

13. _____ Communication: speech impaired. Follows commands well.

14. _____ All other transfers are performed indep & at a functional speed.

PART III. Rewrite the following *O* statements in a more clear, concise, and professional manner. Also, list the subheading under which the statement should be placed. (To assist you, an example is given, and some of the problems are in italics in the first few statements.)

---

example

Passive range of motion is limited to 90 *degrees* of flexion in *both* of her hips.
a. Heading: PROM
b. Corrected statement: Hip flexion limited to 90° bilat

---

1. The *patient* has 4/5 strength in *both* of her *arms*.

  a. Heading: _____

  b. Corrected statement: _____

  _____

2. Performing a *straight leg raise* on the *left reproduces* the *patient's* worst back pain.

  a. Heading: _____

  b. Corrected statement: _____

  _____

3. Strength *is* 5/5 in *right* shoulder *muscles*, 4/5 in *right* biceps, 2/5 in *right* triceps, 0/5 in all other *right* arm musculature distal to the elbow. *Left* arm strength is *normal*.

   a. Heading: _____

   b. Corrected statement: _____

_____

4. *Mary ambulates* for *approximately* 150 *feet full weight bearing with* a walker *twice independently*.

   a. Heading: _____

   b. Corrected statement: _____

_____

5. The patient was short of breath after transferring supine to sit and bed to bedside chair; her respiratory rate increased from 18 breaths per minute before the transfers to 32 breaths per minute immediately after the transfers.

   a. Heading: _____

   b. Corrected statement: _____

_____

6. Left ankle active range of motion is within the normal range.

   a. Heading: _____

   b. Corrected statement: _____

_____

> ■ **PART IV.** The following are the notes to yourself that you jotted down while examining a patient. (While taking notes for yourself, you did not consult Hospital XYZ's approved abbreviations list.)

Cardiovascular OK. Blood Pressure: 110/65, Heart Rate: 75, Resp. Rate: 14.

Integumentary OK.

Musculoskeletal impaired Ⓡ LE.

Neuromuscular impaired gait and locomotion, motor function unimpaired, balance impaired.

Communication age appropriate & unimpaired.

Affect OK.

Cognition unimpaired; oriented—person, place, time.

Learning barriers—none.

Learning style—likes for me to show him prior to him trying to move.

Ed. needs: ambulation with walker and walker safety, transfer safety, protection of cast.

Both UEs—strength & AROM—WNL.

Gait—independent—walker—NWB Ⓛ LE—50 ft. twice.

Ⓛ LE—cast—long leg.

Ⓡ LE AROM normal; strength 5/5 throughout.

Transfers—toilet minimal of 1, sit to and from stand independent, supine to and from sit independent.

Curb—(1-step c̄ walker)—minimal of 1

Ambulates in & out of door—min +1—opens & closes door—walker

Ⓛ LE—not examined further

Rewrite each line into an *O* statement. Include the appropriate subcategory of Systems Review or Tests and Measures before each statement. (Example: Ⓡ UE: AROMs WNL except 90° Ⓡ shoulder flexion.)

1. Cardiovascular OK. Blood Pressure: 110/65, Heart Rate: 75, Resp. Rate: 14

   O statement: _____

   _____

2. Integumentary OK

   O statement: _____

   _____

3. Musculoskeletal impaired Ⓡ LE.

   O statement: _____

   _____

4. Neuromuscular impaired gait and locomotion, motor function unimpaired, balance impaired.

   O statement: _____

   _____

5. Communication age-appropriate & unimpaired.

   O statement: _____

   _____

6. Affect OK

   O statement: _____

   _____

7. Cognition OK; oriented—person, place, time

   O statement: _____

   _____

8. Learning barriers—none

   O statement: _____

   _____

9. Learning style—likes for me to show him prior to him trying to move

   O statement: _____

   _____

10. Ed. needs: ambulation with walker and walker safety, transfer safety, protection of cast

    O statement: _____

    _____

11. Both UEs—strength & AROM—WNL

    O statement: _____

    _____

12. Gait—independent—walker—NWB Ⓛ LE—50 ft. twice

    O statement: _____

    _____

13. Ⓛ LE—cast—long leg

    O statement: _____

    _____

14. Ⓡ LE AROM normal; strength 5/5 throughout

    O statement: _____

    _____

15. Transfers—toilet minimal of 1, sit to and from stand independent, supine to and from sit independent

    O statement: _____

    _____

16. Curb—(1-step c̄ walker)—minimal of 1

    O statement: _____

    _____

17. Ambulates in & out of door—min +1—opens & closes door—walker

    O statement: _____

    _____

18. Ⓛ LE—not assessed further

    O statement: _____

    _____

19. Pt's height is 5 feet 6 in. Weight is 165.

    O statement: _____

    _____

PART V. In the following you will find headings for the *O* portion of a note. Each is followed by blanks (more than are needed for the exercise). Using the statements from Part IV, write the number of each after its appropriate heading. The statements you list after each heading should be in the order in which they would logically appear in a note (for instance, 1–5–3 may make more sense than if you were to order them 3–1–5). Subcategories under Systems Review:

A. Cardiovascular: _____, _____, _____, _____

B. Integumentary: _____, _____, _____, _____

C. Musculoskeletal: _____, _____, _____, _____

D. Neuromuscular: _____, _____, _____, _____

E. Communication: _____, _____, _____, _____

F. Affect: _____, _____, _____, _____

G. Cognition: _____, _____, _____, _____

H. Learning Barriers: _____, _____, _____, _____

I. Learning Style: _____, _____, _____, _____

J. Ed.ucation Needs: _____, _____, _____, _____

Subcategories under Tests and Measures:

K. Amb: _____, _____, _____, _____

L. Transfers: _____, _____, _____, _____

M. UEs & Ⓡ LE: _____, _____, _____, _____

N. Ⓛ LE: _____, _____, _____, _____

PART VI. Using the categories listed previously, use the information to write the *O* portion of a note. (Some of the previous statements may have to be rewritten to combine similar material into a single statement.) Your partial note should be written to be an acceptable part of the patient's medical record at Hospital XYZ (using approved abbreviations).

O: _____

_____

_____

_____

_____

_____

_____

_____

_____

_____

_____

_____

_____

_____

_____

_____

_____

_____

_____

_____

_____

_____

_____

_____

_____

Answers to "Writing Objective (O): Worksheet 1" are provided in Appendix A.

Writing the Objective (O)

> **PART I.** Below you will find headings for the Tests and Measures section of the *O* portion of a note. Each is followed by five blanks (more than are needed for the exercise). Following these headings are statements to be included in the note. Write the number of each after its appropriate subheading. The statements you list after each heading should be in the order in which they would logically appear in a note (for instance, 1–5–3 may make more sense than if you were to order them 3–1–5). You may wish to write the part of the objective section of the note out on a separate piece of paper to assist you with this task.

A. Gait: _____, _____, _____, _____, _____

B. Transfers: _____, _____, _____, _____, _____

C. Ⓡ extremities: _____, _____, _____, _____, _____

D. Ⓛ extremities: _____, _____, _____, _____, _____

1. All transfers are totally dependent.

2. AROM, strength, & sensation to light touch WNL throughout Ⓡ UE & LE.

3. Ⓛ UE & LE very low muscle tone.

4. No active movement noted in Ⓛ extremities.

5. Sensation to light touch intact Ⓛ extremities.

6. Amb not feasible at this time.

7. PROM WNL throughout Ⓛ extremities.

> **PART II.** The following are the notes to yourself that you jotted down during your therapy session while re-examining your patient (for a progress note). (While taking notes for yourself, you did not consult Hospital XYZ's approved abbreviations list.)

Propels w/c himself 15 ft. to mat—difficulty getting close to mat & locking brakes—maximum +1 to place sliding board

Maximum +1 to remove armrest

w/c ↔ mat c̄ sliding board & minimum +1 assist for NWB Ⓡ LE—verbal cues for hand placement

Sit ↔ supine c̄ moderate of 1 to move Ⓡ LE

Hip flex 4/5 Ⓛ, 3−/5 Ⓡ

Hip ext 4/5 Ⓛ, 3/5 Ⓡ

Knee flex 4/5 Ⓛ, 2−/5 Ⓡ

Knee ext 4/5 Ⓛ, 3/5 Ⓡ

Ankle 5/5 bilat all movements

Hip abduction bilaterally at least 3/5 bilat; not tested c̄ resistance against gravity due to patient fatigue

Performed Ⓡ & Ⓛ hip abduction/adduction c̄ 2# ×15 (supine)

Performed Ⓡ & Ⓛ SL Ⓡ ×15 repetitions

Performed knee flex c̄ 2# ×15 repetitions Ⓛ, 1# ×15 repetitions Ⓡ

Performed Ⓛ & Ⓡ terminal knee ext c̄ 2# ×15 repetitions

Requires frequent rests—exercise tolerance low—muscle endurance low

Using the categories of your choice, write the above information into the *O* portion of a progress note. Your partial note should be written to be an acceptable part of the patient's medical record at Hospital XYZ.

O: _____

_____

_____

_____

_____

_____

_____

_____

_____

_____

_____

_____

_____

_____

_____

_____

_____

> **PART III.** Rewrite the following O statements in a more clear, concise, and professional manner. Also, list the heading under which the statement should be placed.

1. The patient walks 50 feet twice with 50 percent partial weight bearing on her left leg and requires verbal cues from me to compensate for her vision deficits.

   a. Heading: _____

   b. Corrected statement: _____

   _____

2. Examination of the patient's left ankle reveals pitting edema.

   a. Heading: _____

   b. Corrected statement: _____

   _____

3. The knee jerk, when tested, is three plus on the right and two plus on the left.

   a. Heading: _____

   b. Corrected statement: _____

   _____

4. John used a sliding board to perform his transfer from the wheelchair to the mat and back, requiring my presence to occasionally provide minimal help to stabilize him when he loses his balance.

   a. Heading: _____

   b. Corrected statement: _____

   _____

5. Mary requires two people using maximal assistance to roll her to either side from lying on her back.

   a. Heading: _____

   b. Corrected statement: _____

   _____

6. Has no learning problems.

   a. Heading: _____

   b. Corrected statement: _____

   _____

Answers to "Writing Objective (O): Worksheet 2" are provided in Appendix A.

Stating the Problem, S & O

> **PART I.** Indicate which of the following statements belong in the *Problem, Subjective,* and *Objective* sections of the SOAP note. Mark them by writing *Prob, S,* or *O* on the blank line before the appropriate statement. (Some of the statements do not belong in these sections of the note.)

1. _____ Incision healing well, length 3 in. location immediately prox. to Ⓛ thumbnail.

2. _____ ↑ AROM Ⓡ shoulder to WNL within 4 wks. c̄ 3×/wk. Rx.

3. _____ Will instruct Pt. in a home exercise program to improve posture & alignment (attached).

4. _____ Pt.'s wife states he amb indep s̄ assist. device PTA.

5. _____ DTRs: normal throughout.

6. _____ Medical Dx: low back pain.

7. _____ Past experience of PT for low back pain s̄ relief of pain.

8. _____ c/o Ⓡ pain in posterolateral aspects of Ⓡ thigh down to the knee; pain intensity: 8 (0 = no pain, 10 = worst possible pain).

9. _____ Will attempt to perform manual muscle test on another date when Pt. is more rested.

10. _____ X-ray: arthritic spurs L3–5 on the Ⓡ .

11. _____ HR 75 ā exercise, 95 immediately p̄ exercise, & 75 bpm 3 min. p̄ exercise.

12. _____ Amb s̄ assist. device indep & s̄ deviations

13. _____ Describes onset of pain immed. s̄ lifting a 50 lb. bag of dog food on 01/01/2008.

14. _____ BID: hot pack to low back for 20 min.

15. _____ Pt.'s rehab. potential is guarded.

> **PART II.** Rewrite the following *Problem, Subjective,* and *Objective* statements in a more clear, concise, and professional manner. Also, list the subsection of the notes (*Problem, Subjective,* or *Objective*) and the heading and subheading, if appropriate, under which the statement should be placed.

1. The patient complains of left lateral knee pain that comes and goes.

   a. <u>Part of the note:</u> _____

   b. <u>Heading (and subheading, if appropriate):</u> _____

   c. <u>Corrected statement:</u> _____

   _____

2. The patient doesn't have as much sensation in the left L5 dermatome.

   a. <u>Part of the note:</u> _____

   b. <u>Heading (and subheading, if appropriate):</u> _____

   c. <u>Corrected statement:</u> _____

   _____

3. The patient states a doctor "looked in [his] right knee with a scope" on 02/02/2008.

   a. <u>Part of the note:</u> _____

   b. <u>Heading (and subheading, if appropriate):</u> _____

   c. <u>Corrected statement:</u> _____

   _____

4. The patient says he had "surgery where they opened up my skull" in February 2008.

   a. <u>Part of the note:</u> _____

   b. <u>Heading (and subheading, if appropriate):</u> _____

   c. <u>Corrected statement:</u> _____

   _____

5. Right leg passive range of motion is within normal limits throughout.

   a. <u>Part of the note:</u> _____

   b. <u>Heading (and subheading, if appropriate):</u> _____

   c. <u>Corrected statement:</u> _____

   _____

> **PART III.** Here are the notes to yourself that you jotted down while reading the chart and examining your patient. (While taking notes for yourself, you did not consult Hospital XYZ's approved abbreviations list.)

FROM THE CHART

Medical diagnosis is fractured right femoral neck on 01/12/2008.

A right hip prosthesis was inserted on 01/13/2008.

Patient is 65 years old.

The patient is male.

Physician is Dr. Sosome.

HgB was 11 this morning.

You are seeing the patient on 01/15/2008.

You tried to see the patient on 01/14/2008 but patient was dizzy lying in bed and HgB was 7.

Patient received blood transfusion on 01/14/2008.

From the Patient

Pain (R) hip while standing 8/10, while lying (before ambulation) 4/10

No PT or OT before—no walker or cane before this admission

No tub chair or portable commode currently available at home—no other assistive devices used for dressing, bathing, ambulating

Ambulation and all activities of daily living were completely independent prior to admission

Fell at home and hit (R) hip on side of bathtub

Lives alone

Lives in senior apartment building—elevator—curbs only

Apartment bathroom has a bathtub with a shower and shower curtain

Retired this year—was a teacher—still volunteers at elementary school 3 days per week, reading with small children

For recreation, patient watches his grandchildren and plays cards with friends. Watches toddler-aged grandchildren once per week and plays cards with friends 2 nights per week

Would like to return to his apartment after discharge

(For PTs:) Would like to eventually ambulate independently s̄ device once again

(For OTs:) Would like to able to manage grooming and dressing by himself; would "settle" for Meals on Wheels

Considers herself in good health

Walks approximately 2 miles 3 times per week

Does not drink alcohol and does not smoke

Pt's parents are in their 90's and are in good health.

States transferred into bedside chair early today and accomplished the transfer with 2 people assisting him

States has had no previous fractures

States has had no hospitalizations prior to the current hospitalization

States takes no medications at home

Systems Review

blood pressure is 120/80

initially pulse rate was 80

respiratory rate was 12

patient is 5 feet 11 inches tall

patient weighs 170 pounds

gait impaired

locomotion impaired

balance impaired in standing and during ambulation

motor function unimpaired

impaired skin at surgery site; otherwise WNL

gross strength impaired on the right as is the range of motion

communication is unimpaired

the patient's emotional/behavioral responses are unimpaired

oriented to person, place, and time; unimpaired

patient wears glasses and cannot read without them—therefore, will need them for the home exercise program

likes to be shown by the therapist and then tries to imitate therapist's actions—visual learner

needs to learn how to use a walker on level surfaces and on curbs, needs to learn transfers, needs to learn to check for proper healing of wound, needs a home exercise program

PT Examination Performed

UEs—ROMs WNL except −5 degrees of right elbow extension

UEs—strength 4+/5 throughout (group muscle test)

ROMs in left leg WNL

Right LE—ROMs limited secondary to post-op restrictions to 90 degrees hip flexion, full active hip abduction, zero degrees hip medial and lateral rotation, 0 degrees adduction

Left LE—strength 4+/5 throughout (group muscle tests)

Right LE—strength at least 3/5 throughout—not further examined due to recent surgery

Transfers   w/c to and from bed c̄ moderate of 1 person

Sit to and from stand with minimal of 1 person

Supine to and from sit with moderate of 1 person

Ambulated—parallel bars minimal of 1 approximately 20 feet once 50% PWB right LE—felt dizzy and nauseated—no further examination or interventions performed this date—nurses notified

BP 145/90 immediately after ambulation, 135/80 3 min. after ambulation

Pulse 105 immediately after ambulation, 82 3 min. after ambulation

Breathing rate 18 immediately after ambulation; 12 3 min. after ambulation

OT Examination Performed

UE strength 4+/5 throughout (group muscle test)

UE—AROM WNL except −5 degrees right elbow extension

Fine motor skills within normal limits

Transfers supine to and from sit with moderate assistance of 1

Transfers wheelchair to and from bed with moderate assistance of 1

Patient able to bathe UE and trunk but needs minimal assistance of 1 for both LEs and needs setup for sponge bath

Able to groom his hair independently

Able to care for his teeth independently

Wears contact lenses; able to care for lenses by himself from a wheelchair

Dressing not assessed this date due to high pain level and low patient endurance

Write the previous information into the *Problem, Subjective,* and *Objective portions* of either a physical therapy note or an occupational therapy note. Your partial note should be written to be an acceptable part of the patient's medical record at Hospital XYZ.

_____

_____

_____

_____

_____

_____

_____

_____

_____

_____

_____

_____

_____

_____

_____

_____

_____

_____

_____

_____

_____

_____

_____

_____

_____

_____

_____

_____

_____

_____

Answers to Review Worksheet: Stating the Problem, S, and O can be found in Appendix A.

III | Documenting the Evaluation (A)

*A*fter a health care professional performs an examination, the next step is the process of making clinical decisions. This process includes listing the patient's areas of deficit at the impairment, functional, and disability levels, as well as listing the relationship among the patient's areas of deficit. This process also includes determining the patient's diagnosis and prognosis. Part III of this book covers the Evaluation (Chapter 11), Diagnosis (Chapter 12), and Prognosis (Chapter 13) parts of the note. This is the portion of managing the patient/client that only therapists perform.

The Patient/Client Management Note has three sections called *Evaluation, Diagnosis,* and *Prognosis.* In the SOAP Note, the Evaluation, Diagnosis, and Prognosis parts of the note are listed in a section called the *Assessment.* In some facilities, the expected outcomes and anticipated goals are listed in the Assessment part of the note.

11 | Writing the Evaluation (A: EVALUATION)

*A*fter the therapist completes the examination, the process of evaluation begins. The therapist reviews the History, Systems Review, and Tests and Measures (or Problem, S, and O) parts of the note to capture all of the functional deficits and impairments. These functional deficits and impairments are then listed. After listing the functional deficits and impairments, the therapist explains the relationship among the impairments, functional deficits, and disability levels, when appropriate.

example

Pt. has functional deficits in the areas of ambulation c̄ a walker on level surfaces and stairs, transfers sit ↔ stand, supine ↔ sit, & on/off toilet. Pt.'s functional deficits correspond to the Pt.'s NWB Ⓛ LE status & the impairments of ↓ strength of Ⓡ LE & bilat. UE musculature &

a ↓ in exercise tolerance & muscle endurance. An ↑ in muscle strength & endurance & exercise tolerance should lead to an ↑ in function. Therefore, exercises for strengthening Ⓡ LE & bilat. UE musculature & functional activities should lead to an ↑ in strength, muscle endurance, exercise tolerance, & function.

Importance of the Evaluation Section of the Note

The Evaluation section of the note is a reflection of the therapist's clinical judgments. It often includes a summary of the deficits in function and impairments

115

listed in the previous sections of the note. This summary is useful to other health care providers who want to read a brief summary of the deficits noted in the note. This assists those providers to locate deficits listed in the sections above the Evaluation section of the note.[1,2] Also, third-party payors can review this section of the note to obtain a summary of deficits and the relationship between functional deficits and impairments.

The evaluation section also decribes relationships between functional deficits and impairments. These functional deficits and impairments combined with the patient's environment may determine a patient's level of disability in that environment. New or chronic conditions that influence the patient's rate of recovery are also described in this section of the note. Reasons for referral may also be in this section of the note.[1,2]

Describing Relationships and Justifying Decisions

The Evaluation section of the note provides an opportunity for the therapist to describe the relationships between the examination findings that would not necessarily be obvious to all parties who read patient care notes. It should describe how impairments relate to the functional deficits and how these functional deficits keep the patient from functioning in his or her specific environment.

> example
>
> ↓ Ⓡ shoulder AROM is preventing Pt. from reaching into overhead cabinets. This prevents Pt. from taking care of herself in her home. Ⓡ knee ↓AROM is preventing Pt. from becoming indep. in amb. c̄ walker & in coming sit ↔ stand. Pt. cannot return to her prior status of living alone in the community until she is able to amb. s̄ walker & transfer sit ↔ indep.

Justification for Further Therapy

The Prognosis portion of the note could also include justification for further therapy for a patient who initially appears relatively independent with one functional activity.

> example
>
> Although amb is indep, Pt.'s progress toward indep transfers is slow but steady, possibly due to Pt.'s advanced age. Pt. cont. to need assist. & will benefit from further therapy to work toward indep transfers.

Discussion of Patient's Progress in Therapy

A discussion of the patient's progress in therapy could include further explanation of the patient's failure to progress as quickly as the goals predicted. It could also explain why a patient suddenly regresses or progresses more quickly than anticipated.

> example
>
> Pt. has become more dependent in transfers during the past 2 wks. 2° inactivity associated with patient's recent medical dx of pneumonia.

Inconsistencies

In the Evaluation portion of the note, the therapist has the opportunity to pinpoint inconsistencies between examination findings.

> example
>
> Although patient states entire Ⓛ LE is so painful that it inhibits normal walking, patient amb. over 500 ft. on treadmill FWB s̄ assist. device & s̄ gait deviations.

Further Testing Needed

Tests and measures that would be helpful but could not be completed during the initial therapy session can be listed. The therapist can also list the plans for further tests and measures.

> example
>
> Further testing of sensation & proprioception is needed & will be performed within 1 wk.

Referral to Another Practitioner

Reasons for referral to another practitioner may be discussed in this section. The reasons for referral are often a result of the screening done in the Systems Review. Sometimes, information combined from the Systems Review and Tests and Measures leads to referral to another health care provider.

As the therapist performs an examination, if the examination findings do not fall within the scope of therapy practice, the therapist refers the patient to other practitioners who are educated to intervene appropriately with those findings. Physicians refer to other practitioners, including therapists, to intervene more specifically with patient problems that fall within the scope of therapy practice.

> example
>
> Examination revealed ↑ size of lymph nodes inferior to the Ⓛ clavicle. Examination & evaluation by a physician is indicated. Pt. referred to her primary care physician for medical examination and evaluation of Ⓛ subclavicular area.

Summary and Objective

The Evaluation section of the note is very important for the therapist. This is the section of the note in which deficits in function and impairments are listed. This section of the note explains the relationships between impairments and function, the rationale for referral to another clinician, and the rationale for the therapist's decision to delay a type of examination or to examine the patient using an alternative method. The worksheets for this chapter follow Chapter 13. After reviewing the previous information, completing all of the worksheets, and comparing your work to the answer sheets, you should be able to write the Evaluation portion of the note with assistance in making connections between examination results and the patient's ability to function in his or her environment.

References

1. American Physical Therapy Association: Guide to Physical Therapist Practice, ed. 2, and CD-ROM. American Physical Therapy Association, Alexandria, VA, 2003.
2. American Physical Therapy Association: Defensible Documentation for Patient/Client Management. Accessed at http://www.apta.org/AM/ Template.cfm?Section= Documentation4&Template=/MembersOnly. cfm&ContentID=37776 on March 9, 2007.

12 Writing the Diagnosis (A: DIAGNOSIS)

As discussed in Chapter 11, after the therapist completes the examination, the process of evaluation begins. As part of the evaluative process, the therapist looks at the patient's functional deficits and impairments discussed in the evaluation section of the note, and places them in a diagnostic category, or practice pattern, as listed in *The Guide to Physical Therapist Practice*.[1] The therapist also looks at more specific movement dysfunction categories that fit under the practice pattern and may more specifically describe the patient's functional deficits and impairments by describing the patient's condition using one or more of those categories.[1,2] This diagnostic process is another process involved in managing the patient/client that only therapists perform.

Differences Between a Therapy Diagnosis and a Medical Diagnosis

A diagnosis by a therapist describes the impact that functional deficits or impairments have on the person's ability to function in his or her environment. These are the functional deficits or impairments toward which the therapists direct therapy interventions. A medical diagnosis uses categories to describe medical signs and symptoms and directs medical interventions toward these signs and symptoms.

> **example**
>
> Pt. has hx of diabetes & prior Ⓛ foot ulcers, ↓ ROM & strength Ⓛ foot & ankle, shoes c̄ orthotics that do not fit, ↓ sensation Ⓛ foot, placing Pt.'s condition in Integumentary Pattern A: Primary Prevention/Risk Reduction for Integumentary Disorders.

Secondary Practice Patterns/ Movement Dysfunctions

At times, the patient may have multiple functional deficits or impairments that could place the patient in more than one practice pattern or diagnostic category. In these cases, it is appropriate to list the secondary practice patterns or diagnostic category(-ies) and explain the rationale for the listing of practice patterns as primary or secondary. It is also appropriate to discuss the progression of a patient from one diagnostic pattern to another, as needed.

> **example**
>
> <u>Primary diagnostic category</u> on this date is Cardiovascular/Pulmonary Pattern C: Impaired Ventilation, Respiration/Gas Exchange, & Aerobic Capacity/Endurance Associated with Airway Clearance Dysfunction in response to the medical dx of Ⓡ lower lobe pneumonia. <u>Secondary diagnostic category</u> is Musculoskeletal Pattern G: Impaired Joint Mobility, Muscle Performance and Range of Motion Associated with Fx that correlates with the medical dx of fx Ⓡ femoral neck. As pneumonia clears, Musculoskeletal Pattern G will become the 1° practice pattern.

Alternative Diagnostic Schemes

As further diagnostic paradigms develop, it is appropriate for the therapist to list both the diagnostic category(-ies) listed in the *Guide to Physical Therapist Practice*[1] and a more specific diagnosis made by the therapist from a diagnostic model. For the purposes of this text, you will be expected to list the diagnostic category(s) from the *Guide to Physical Therapist Practice*[1] with guidance.

Use of ICD-9 Codes

In some facilities, therapists select the ICD-9 CM code most closely associated with the patient's diagnosis. These codes are used for billing purposes. If the therapist selects an ICD-9CM code, it may be listed in the Diagnosis section of the note.[2] For the purposes of this book, you will not be asked to list an ICD-9 Code in the Diagnosis section of the note.

Summary and Objective

The Diagnosis portion of the Patient/Client Management Note or the SOAP Note is extremely important. It places the patient's functional deficits and impairments into a practice pattern and may identify a more specific movement dysfunction category. The Diagnosis part of the note, as a whole, requires much professional judgment. Experience will enable the new practitioner to write this section of the note more easily and without assistance.

The worksheets that follow Chapter 13 will give you practice writing the Evaluation, Diagnosis, and Prognosis sections of a patient care note. After reviewing the previous information, completing all of the worksheets, and comparing your work to the answer sheets, you should be able to write the Diagnosis section of the note with assistance in identifying the specific practice pattern from the *Guide to Physical Therapist Practice*.[1]

References

1. American Physical Therapy Association: Guide to Physical Therapist Practice, ed. 2, and CD-ROM. American Physical Therapy Association, Alexandria, VA, 2003.
2. American Physical Therapy Association: Defensible Documentation for Patient/Client Management. Accessed at http://www.apta.org/AM/ Template.cfm?Section=Documentation4&Template=/MembersOnly.cfm&ContentID=37776 on March 9, 2007.

13 | Writing the Prognosis

After the therapist completes the examination and determines a therapy diagnosis, the therapist then determines a prognosis. The therapist looks at the severity of the patient's functional deficits and impairments, the patient goals, and living environment, and predicts a level of improvement in function and the amount of time needed to reach the level. This is part of the patient/client management process that only therapists perform. As part of a discussion of the prognosis, several kinds of information may be addressed. Each category of information is briefly described in the following text.[1,2]

Factors Influencing the Prognosis

A discussion of factors influencing the prognosis such as living environment, patient's condition prior to the onset of the current therapy diagnosis, and current illnesses or medical conditions may be included.

> **example**
>
> With current medical dx of CA, Pt.'s poor functioning in the home PTA, & the stairs the Pt. must amb. daily at home, return to home alone is not a safe alternative.

Justification for the Goals Set, the Treatment Plan, and/or Clarification of the Problem

The Prognosis part of a note might include a statement justifying unusual goals. For example, a therapist might get a patient with a diagnosis of stroke who has the potential to transfer independently. However, the patient's wife has been helping to transfer him for years. Both he and his wife are satisfied with the situation and do not want to change the way they have been living. You might then set your goal, "Pt. will perform all transfers c̄ min assist. from his wife within 1 mo." You would comment, "A goal of indep transfers is not realistic due to Pt.'s previous functional level of requiring assist. for transfers from his wife, & Pt. & wife's desire to return to the previous functional level only."

Future Services Needed

Community services that would be helpful to the patient or may be helpful to the patient in the future can be discussed.

> **example**
>
> Pt. would benefit from home health physical therapy p̄ D/C from the hospital.

Summary and Objective

The Prognosis portion of the Patient/Client Management Note or the SOAP Note is an important part of the note that documents the therapist's professional opinion about the level of improvement that may be attained.

The worksheets that follow this chapter will give you practice writing the Evaluation, Diagnosis, and Prognosis.

After reviewing the previous information, completing all of the worksheets, and comparing your work to the answer sheets, you should be able to write the Prognosis portion of the note with assistance in identifying the level of improvement that the patient may reach and time frames that may be required to reach that level.

References

1. American Physical Therapy Association: Guide to Physical Therapist Practice, ed. 2, and CD-ROM. American Physical Therapy Association, Alexandria, VA, 2003.
2. American Physical Therapy Association: Defensible Documentation for Patient/Client Management. Accessed at http://www.apta.org/AM/ Template.cfm?Section= Documentation4&Template=/MembersOnly. cfm&ContentID=37776 on March 9, 2007.

Writing the Evaluation, Diagnosis, and Prognosis

> ■ **PART I.** Mark the statements that should be placed in the Evaluation part of the note by writing *Eval.* on the line before the statement. Mark the statements that should be placed in the Diagnosis part of the note by writing *Diag.* on the line before the statement. Mark the statements that should be placed in the Prognosis part of the note by writing *Prog.* on the line before the statement. Some statements will not belong in the Evaluation, Diagnosis, or Prognosis part of the note. Also mark the History statements with an *Hx*, the Systems Review statements with *SR*, and the Tests and Measures statements by writing *T & M* on the blank line before the statement.

1. _TM_____ Strength: Grossly 2/5 throughout all extremities.

2. _SR_____ Musculoskeletal System: Gross strength impaired all extremities.

3. _Hx_____ C/o pain ⓡ knee of intensity of 6 on a 0–10 scale (0 = no pain; 10 = worst possible pain).

4. _Hx_____ States gradual onset of pain in [month, year].

5. _Hx_____ Pt. states healing process of residual limb was slowed by infection; took 5 months to heal.

6. _____ Indep. in donning/doffing prosthesis within 1 wk. to enable the Pt. to become indep. in amb.

7. _Diag._____ Will discuss referral to a dietitian c̄ Pt.'s physician. →diagnose that it's not in your realm of practice.

8. _____ ↑ AROM ⓡ shoulder to WNL within 6 wks. to enable Pt. to reach items in her overhead cabinets.

9. _Prog._____ Pt.'s weight will cause progress in PT to be somewhat slow; anticipate a course of therapy for 8 weeks 3×/wk. as an OP.

10. _~~Prog.~~/Hx_ Medical dx: B/K amputation ⓡ LE.

11. _~~SR~~ Hx_ Pt. has been confined to a w/c while residual limb healing occurred.

12. _Hx_____ Pt. goals: To return home s̄ assist. p̄ 1 wk. of Rx BID

13. _Prog._____ Pt. is young & had a high level of function prior to amputation; therefore, rehab. prognosis is good.

14. _TM_____ PROM: WNL bilat. LEs.

15. _~~Rx~~ SR_ Learning barriers: very hard of hearing; does not wear hearing aid.

16. _____ Pulsed US underwater at 1.5–2.0 W/cm² to ⓡ wrist.

17. _____ Medical hx of TIA in 2006, ASHD, CHF.

18. _Prog._____ Rehab. prognosis guarded. Pt.'s prior level of function was low. Return to prior level of function will be difficult c̄ further deconditioning 2° prolonged bedrest.

19. _Diag._____ Practice pattern Musculoskeletal J: Impaired Motor Function, Muscle Performance, ROM, Gait, Locomotion, & Balance Associated c̄ Amputation.

20. _Prog._____ Pt. will progress much more quickly p̄ Pt. is allowed to be FWB ⓛ LE.

21. _Hx_____ States hx of COPD since 2007.

22. _TM_____ Hip clearing reproduces pain ⓛ knee.

TIA =

US = ultra sound

ASHD =

CHF =

PART II. Determine which of the following statements should be placed in the Evaluation part of the note, which should be placed in the Diagnosis part of the note, and which should be placed in the Prognosis part of the note. Mark the statements that should be placed in the Evaluation part of the note by writing *Eval.* on the line before the statement. Mark the statements that should be placed in the Diagnosis part of the note by writing *Diag.* on the line before the statement. Mark the statements that should be placed in the Prognosis part of the note by writing *Prog.* on the line before the statement.

1. _____ Pt.'s c/o fall outside of the practice area of physical therapy. Contacted Pt.'s physician and Pt. was sent to the Emergency Room for immediate attention.

2. _____ Rehab. potential is good; will progress quickly to independence.

3. _____ Pt. will need Home Health PT p̄ D/C from the hospital to cont. toward indep. on steps. Pt. must amb. at home.

4. _____ ↓ Ⓡ ankle AROM is related to Pt.'s gait deviations. Gait deviations are preventing Pt. from returning to indep. amb. in the community s̄ assist. device. Pt. is required to be indep. s̄ assist. device to return to work.

5. _____ Prognosis is good for complete rehab; however, progress will be slowed by Pt.'s medical dx of COPD.

6. _____ Pt.'s case is most consistent with Practice Pattern G Impaired Joint Mobility, Muscle Performance, & Range of Motion Associated with Fracture.

PART III. Rewrite the following statements into the Evaluation, Diagnosis, and Prognosis parts of the note.

1. The results of the examination reveal that the patient's condition fits into two categories: Musculoskeletal pattern G for the patient's fx Ⓛ radius and ulna and Neuromuscular pattern D for the stroke with left-sided hemiplegia. Musculoskeletal Pattern G = Impaired Joint Mobility, Muscle Performance, & ROM Associated With Fracture. Neuromuscular Pattern D = Impaired Motor Function & Sensory Integrity Associated With Nonprogressive Disorders of the Central Nervous System—Acquired in Adolescence or Adulthood. You believe that the primary practice pattern is Neuromuscular Pattern D because the deficits involved are greater, such as significant gait deviations, need to use an assistive device in gait with assistance, and inability to use the left arm in a functional manner. You believe the patient has good rehabilitation potential. She is relatively young, motivated, cooperative, and cognitively sound. The inability to use her left arm in a functional manner is affecting her ability to perform ADLs, and her gait deviations and need for assistance in ambulating with an assistive device prevent her from functioning at home independently and from doing her work as a cashier outside of the home.

_____

_____

_____

_____

_____

_____

_____

_____

_____

_____

2. After performing an examination, you determine that your patient fits into Musculoskeletal Pattern J: Impaired Joint Mobility, Motor Function, Muscle Performance, and Range of Motion Associated With Amputation. The patient has had an amputation below the knee; on the right. You believe the patient's rehabilitation potential is fair because the patient has a medical diagnosis of Alzheimer's Disease. The patient lives on an Alzheimer's Unit in a nursing home. The patient follows simple commands, and you believe the patient could become functional at transferring bed↔w/c with minimal assistance and verbal cues. This would assist the nursing home staff in caring for the patient (decrease risk to his caretakers), would maximize his activity level and quality of life, and would further prevent any pulmonary and integumentary problems. The patient's decreased function in transfers is impairing his ability to participate in activities in the nursing home and is placing the health of the nursing home staff at risk.

Answers to "Writing Evaluation, Diagnosis and Prognosis: Worksheet 1" are provided in Appendix A.

Writing the Evaluation, Diagnosis, and Prognosis

> ■ **PART I.** Mark the statements that should be placed in the Evaluation part of the note by writing *Eval.* on the line before the statement. Mark the statements that should be placed in the Diagnosis part of the note by writing *Diag.* on the line before the statement. Mark the statements that should be placed in the Prognosis part of the note by writing *Prog.* on the line before the statement. Some statements will belong in neither the Diagnosis nor Prognosis part of the note. Also mark the Problem statements with *Prob.*, the Subjective statements with *S*, and the Objective statements with *O* on the blank line before the statement.

1. _____ States was in a car accident & Pt. was thrown from car.

2. _____ Indep. walker amb. 150 ft. ×2 FWB within 2 wks. to allow Pt. to amb. from her car into her house.

3. _____ Cognition: Pt. is not oriented to date, place, or task & does not follow instructions consistently.

4. _____ Transfers: Supine ↔ sit c̄ min. + 1 assist.

5. _____ Proprioception: ↓ noted throughout entire ⓇLE.

6. _____ Will see BID at B/S.

7. _____ Musculoskeletal practice pattern H: Impaired Joint Mobility, Motor Function, Muscle Performance, & ROM Associated c̄ Joint Arthroplasty.

8. _____ c/o inability to dress indep.

9. _____ Hx of osteoarthritis since 2008.

10. _____ DTRs 2+ throughout LEs except 3+ Ⓡ KJ noted.

11. _____ ↓ ROM & strength Ⓡ LE are associated c̄ Pt.'s gait deviations & dependence in amb. Gait deviations & dependence in amb. prevent Pt. from functioning indep. at home.

12. _____ Learning style: Pt. prefers to watch a demonstration ā attempting a new activity; visual learner.

13. _____ c/o pain in "entire" Ⓛ LE c̄ active or passive movement of Ⓛ knee.

14. _____ Pt. has excellent rehab. potential.

15. _____ Pt. will need 1–2 home health care visits to teach Pt. to amb. steps at home.

16. _____ Sensation: Absent to light touch & pinprick throughout C5 distribution.

17. _____ Gross strength impaired Ⓛ LE.

18. _____ 2° practice pattern is Integumentary Pattern C: Impaired Integumentary Integrity Associated With Partial-Thickness Skin Involvement & Scar Formation.

19. _____ Pt. has partial-thickness open wound plantar surface of Ⓛ foot on 1st MP joint 1 cm × 0.8 cm in size.

20. _____ Amb. will progress quickly once Ⓛ foot is healed.

PART II. Determine which of the following statements should be placed in the Evaluation part of the note, which should be placed in the Diagnosis part of the note and which should be placed in the Prognosis part of the note. Mark the statements that should be placed in the Evaluation part of the note by writing *Eval.* on the line before the statement. Mark the statements that should be placed in the Diagnosis part of the note by writing *Diag.* on the line before the statement. Mark the statements that should be placed in the Prognosis part of the note by writing *Prog.* on the line before the statement.

---

1. _____ Pt.'s rehab. potential is poor. Pt. did not cooperate with initial examination 2° cognitive confusion.

2. _____ Will refer to social services to assist. Pt.'s daughter c̄ appropriate ways to deal c̄ the Pt.'s obstinate behavior.

3. _____ Cardiovascular/Pulmonary Practice Pattern A: Primary Prevention/Risk Reduction for Cardiovascular/Pulmonary Disorders.

4. _____ Pt. could benefit from PT in the nursing home to which she is transferring. Pt. needs work on indep. & safe amb.

5. _____ ↑ muscle spasm in lumbar paraspinal musculature, ↓ trunk ROM & ↓ ability to tolerate sitting is causing Pt. to spend ↓ hrs. at work.

PART III. Rewrite the following statements into the Diagnosis and Prognosis parts of the note.

---

1. The results of the examination reveal that the patient's condition falls into the Musculoskeletal practice pattern G for the patient's fx Ⓡ radius and ulna. Musculoskeletal Pattern G = Impaired Joint Mobility, Muscle Performance, & ROM Associated with Fracture. The patient's decreased ROM and strength in the Ⓡ wrist are causing the patient to have difficulty c̄ ADLs such as eating & writing. The patient's work involves typing for more than 50% of the time & she is currently unable to type s̄ pain. You believe that the patient has good rehabilitation potential. You believe the patient should progress well with PT because she is active and follows instructions well.

_____

_____

_____

_____

_____

_____

_____

_____

_____

_____

_____

_____

_____

_____

_____

2. The patient's right extremity strength, motor planning, and mobility impairments will prevent the patient from returning home alone. The patient will need to regain independent ambulation and ADLs to return home. The results of the examination reveal that the patient falls into the Neuromuscular Practice Pattern D: Impaired Motor Function & Sensory Integrity Associated c̄ Nonprogressive Disorders of the CNS—Acquired in Adolescence or Adulthood. The patient's rehabilitation potential is fair. The patient may need prolonged time to regain movement of her left extremities & overall mobility because of her advanced age.

Answers to "Writing Evaluation, Diagnosis and Prognosis: Worksheet 2" are provided in Appendix A.

History, Systems Review, Tests & Measures, Evaluation, Diagnosis, Prognosis (Problem, S, O, A)

Begin by turning to the corresponding answer sheets at the end of these instructions so that you can write your partial Patient/Client Management and SOAP Notes directly on the answer sheet.

The following are notes to yourself that you jotted down while reading the chart, interviewing, and performing a systems review and tests and measures on your patient. (While taking notes for yourself, you did not consult Hospital XYZ's approved abbreviations list nor were you particularly careful in your notation style.)

1. Write the information into the *History, Systems Review, and Tests and Measures* parts of a Patient/Client Management Note. (Further instructions will be provided to help you write the *Evaluation, Diagnosis, and Prognosis* parts of the note.) Your partial note should be written to be an acceptable part of the patient's medical record at Hospital XYZ.

2. Write the information into the *Problem, S, O, and A* parts of a SOAP Note. Your partial note should be written to be an acceptable part of the patient's medical record at Hospital XYZ.

 ## FROM THE MEDICAL RECORD

The medical diagnosis is degenerative joint disease ⓇR hip—total hip replacement performed on [date]
History of htn
Takes [antihypertensive medication]
65 y.o. male
Dr. Sienn
One prior hospitalization—for Left total hip replacement 01/10/2007

From the Interview

ⓇR hip pain—area of sutures—intensity of 7 when moving—intensity of 3 when sitting (0 = no pain, 10 = worst possible pain)—intensity of 2 when lying still
Prior to adm.—intensity of pain was 9 or 10 and pain was constant
1 step at home to get into the house—railing on ⓇR going up
Owns a 3-in-1 commode, a walker, and a cane
Previous left total hip replacement 01/10/2007
Immediately prior to admission—no assistive device
Lives w/ wife—in his own home
Retired—hobby is gardening
Plans to return home with his wife after D/C
Eventually wants to return to gardening and yard work activities
Does not recall precautions for patients with total hip replacements
Does volunteer ushering at church—also does gardening outside of the church
Right-hand dominant
Does not smoke; only occasionally drinks ETOH
Tried to walk for exercise daily—only ambulated one block prior to admission; two years ago ambulated a mile or more
Rates general health as good
Has had no major life changes in the past year

Pt.'s father died of MI at age 78
Pt.'s mother died of breast cancer at age 72
Pt. has no siblings

Systems Review

Cardiovascular/pulmonary: not impaired
HR: 80
Resp. rate: 14
BP: 130/85
Edema: none noted
Integumentary: impaired
Disruption: staples Ⓡ hip
Continuity of skin color: WNL
Skin texture: not tested this date
Musculoskeletal system:
Gross symmetry: not impaired
Gross ROM: impaired Ⓡ hip and knee
Gross Strength: impaired Ⓡ hip and knee
Height: 6 ft. 0 in.
Weight: 185 pounds
Neuromuscular system:
Gait: impaired
Locomotion: impaired transfers and bed mobility
Balance: impaired in standing—uses walker; not impaired in sitting
Motor function: not impaired
Communication: not impaired
Cognition: oriented ×3; not impaired
Learning barriers: wears glasses—cannot read w/o glasses
Education needs: home exercise program, precautions for patients with total hip replacement, progression of
    recovery process, use of walker, ADLs, including transfers
Learning style: demonstration, then trying an activity

From the Tests & Measures Performed

Sit to/from stand w/ moderate of 1
Supine to and from sit with minimal of 1
W/c to/from mat pivot with moderate of 1
Toilet transfers not tested this date due to decreased activity tolerance of Pt. this date
UE AROM WNL
UE strength 4+/5 throughout bilaterally (group muscle test)
Ⓛ LE strength 4/5 throughout (individual muscle testing performed)
Ⓛ LE AROM WNL throughout
Right LE—strength grossly 1/5 in hip and knee musculature—ankle dorsiflexion 4+/5—ankle plantar flexion at
    least 2/5 but not tested further because of the restricted weight bearing status
Right LE—AROM—WNL ankle—PROM 0–20° hip flexion, 0–10° hip abduction, 0° hip extension—adduction of
    hip, medial and lateral rotation not tested because of hip precautions and recent surgery—knee: 0–70°
Incision— Ⓡ hip—10 cm long—staples intact—over greater trochanter right
Stood bedside with walker moderate of 1 for 1 minute twice—10% PWB right LE

Writing the Evaluation, Diagnosis, and Prognosis

Your opinion is that independent ambulation with a walker is necessary for the patient to go home with a walker. Impairments of decreased ROM and strength right LE are associated with dependent ambulation on this date.

The patient fits into Practice Pattern Musculoskeletal H: Impaired Joint Mobility, Motor Function, Muscle Performance & ROM Associated With Joint Arthroplasty.

The patient has good rehabilitation potential. His level of function was good prior to admission and he has a great desire to return to a healthy, active lifestyle in the community. The patient should be able to return to home with his wife independent in ambulation and a home exercise program to continue to increase right LE strength and ROM after 2-3 days of therapy BID.

PART I. Use this answer sheet to write the *History, Systems Review, Tests and Measures, Evaluation, Diagnosis, and Prognosis* parts of a Patient/Client Management Note.

PART II. Use this answer sheet to write the *Problem, S, O, and A* parts of a SOAP Note.

_____

_____

_____

_____

_____

_____

_____

_____

_____

_____

_____

_____

_____

_____

_____

_____

_____

_____

_____

Answers to "Review Worksheet: History, Systems Review, Tests & Measures, Evaluation, Diagnosis, Prognosis (Problem, S, O, A) are provided in Appendix A.

IV Documenting the Plan of Care (P)

*A*fter a health care professional performs the Examination and Evaluation process, the next step is determining the Plan of Care. This process includes writing Expected Outcomes and Anticipated Goals for the patient and planning interventions to help the patient achieve the expected outcomes and anticipated goals. Part IV of Writing Patient/Client Notes covers the Expected Outcomes (Chapter 14), Anticipated Goals (Chapter 15), and Intervention Plan (Chapter 16) parts of the note.

The Patient/Client Management Note has three sections of the Plan of Care called *Expected Outcomes, Anticipated Goals,* and *Intervention Plan.* In the SOAP Note, the Expected Outcomes, Anticipated Goals, and Intervention Plan parts of the note are listed in a section called Plan of Care (P).

14 Writing Expected Outcomes (Long-Term Goals)

*T*he Plan of Care part of the note is the same for both the Patient/Client Management Note and the SOAP Note. It contains a section of Expected Outcomes, a section of Anticipated Goals, and an Intervention Plan that includes Discharge Plans. Many facilities provide a place for the patient or family member to sign the Plan of Care as proof of informed consent.

The Expected Outcomes section describes the final product to be achieved by therapy. After completing the examination and evaluation, including the process of evaluation, diagnosis, and prognosis, the therapist sets Expected Outcomes. These outcomes are listed in terms of function.[1,2] This chapter addresses the process of writing Expected Outcomes.

Reasons for Writing Expected Outcomes

Expected Outcomes are written for several reasons. These reasons include:

1. to help the therapist plan interventions to meet the specific needs and problems of the patient,
2. to set priorities between interventions and measure the effectiveness of the interventions,
3. to assist with monitoring cost effectiveness (for purposes of third-party payment),
4. to communicate the therapy goals for the patient to other health care professionals.

The Structure of Outcomes and Goals

Before writing Expected Outcomes specifically, it is necessary to know the ABCs of writing objectives. Like an educational objective, a good outcome or goal for patient care contains the following four elements:

A. Audience (who will exhibit the skill)
B. Behavior (what the person will do)
C. Condition (what circumstances—the position, the equipment, and so forth—must be provided or be available for the person to perform the behavior)
D. Degree (how well the behavior will be done—number of feet, number of times performed, amount of assistance needed [i.e., the amount of improvement you want to see specifically] and by when the outcome will be achieved)[3]

Audience

Almost always, the patient is the audience.[3] However, it can be a family member or the patient with a family member, as in "Pt. c̄ his wife will be indep. in amb. stairs & curbs s̄ assist. device." Often the audience is implied in writing outcomes or goals, and it is not necessary to say "Pt. will demonstrate..." or "Pt. will be..."

The audience is *never* the therapist. Outcomes are patient-oriented, not therapist-oriented.

Behavior

The behavior is always an action verb, often followed by the object of the behavior. In the case of writing outcomes, this is a functional behavior. The object of the behavior must be something that can be *measured* or *described accurately* so that you can document when these outcomes are achieved.[3] An example is "Pt. will demonstrate head control in all planes during eating 100% of the time." (Behavior: demonstrate; object of the behavior: head control during eating.)

Sometimes the behavior is implied and not specifically stated. For example, "Indep. *amb & transfers* to provide Pt. indep. mobility within his home." (Unstated behavior: demonstrate; object of the behavior: ambulation & transfers.)

Behaviors are always stated using *action verbs*. Verbs such as *be, know,* or *understand* do not describe observable or measurable activities and, therefore, are not acceptable. Instead, verbs such as *demonstrate, list, state,* and *explain* are acceptable.[3]

Condition

Condition includes the circumstances under which the behavior must be done or the conditions necessary for the behavior to occur.[3] An example is "Indep. *walker* amb. *on level surfaces & curbs* for over 500 ft. ×4 within 3 wks. to allow Pt. indep. mobility at home." A walker, level surfaces, and curbs must be available for the patient to perform this type of ambulation. Another example is

"Pt. will demonstrate head control in all planes during eating 100% of the time." The patient must be eating to fulfill this outcome.

Degree

Degree is usually the longest portion of the Expected Outcomes. It includes the minimal number (example: 40 ft.), the percentage or proportion (example: 3/4 times or 100% of the time), any limitation or departure from a fixed standard (example: Pt. and his wife will indep. navigate stairs with a walker), or any distinguishing features of successful performance (example: Pt. will indep. don/doff prosthesis, choosing appropriate sock thickness for correct fit).

When writing outcomes, the degree of performance must be *realistic, measurable,* or *observable;* must name a specific *time span* in which the outcome will be achieved; and must be *expressed in terms of function.* Discussion of the inclusion of functional terms and the setting of a time span follows.[3]

Notice the example of an outcome given previously: "Indep walker amb. on level surfaces & curbs *for over 500 feet* ×4 (measurable) *within 3 wks.* (time span) *to allow Pt. indep. mobility at home* (functional terms)."

An analysis of all of the parts of the same Expected Outcome follows: "Indep. walker amb. on level surfaces & curbs for over 500 ft. ×4 within 3 wks. to allow Pt. indep. mobility at home."

A. Pt.
B. will amb. (demonstrate ambulation)
C. walker (must be present)
   on level surfaces & curbs (these surfaces must be available)
D. for over 500 ft. ×4 (measurable)
   Indep. (observable)
   within 3 wks. (time span)
   to allow Pt. indep. mobility at home (functional)

Another example is "Pt. will be able to reach shelves in overhead cabinets at least 6 ft. 6 in. above the floor indep. & s̄ pain within 3 wks. to allow Pt. to be able to perform kitchen tasks at home."

A. Pt.
B. will be able to reach into overhead cabinets
C. it is assumed that overhead with shelves at least 6 ft. 6 in. above the floor are present
D. indep. (observable)
   at least 6 ft. 6 in. above the floor (measurable)
   s̄ pain (measurable if you ask Pt. to rate pain on a pain scale)
   within 3 wks. (time span)
   to allow Pt. to be able to perform kitchen tasks at home (functional)

Functional Terms

Some facilities do not add the final phrase to the outcome to put it in functional terms. The advantage of using the final phrase in the previous examples is to notify third-party payors of the functional reasons for the goal. Although it may seem apparent that ambulation and reaching into overhead cabinets are useful tasks for home, this is not always so clear to others.

It is essential that the Expected Outcomes of therapy are stated in functional terms because the ultimate goal of therapy is to make the patient more functional.[2]

Time Span

Expected Outcomes are the functional goals for the patient that have a time span of a week, a month, a year, or longer, depending on the patient's diagnosis, medical history, and general condition.[2] The time span set is the total length of time during which the Pt. will be seen in therapy.[2] For example, in an acute-care setting, a patient may be seen for only 3 to 5 days, but the patient may also be seen in home health care and/or outpatient therapy in order to meet the outcomes of therapy.

Setting the Time Span. Setting a specific time span for your Expected Outcomes is difficult, especially for the new practitioner, because it takes clinical experience to know how quickly a patient will progress. Even experienced therapists cannot always accurately predict the amount of time needed to achieve an outcome. Remember, Expected Outcomes can be revised if your patient cannot reach the outcomes within the time span set. *The Guide to Physical Therapist Practice*[1] gives some general guidelines for number of visits, but patients may have secondary therapy diagnoses or medical diagnoses that cause the patient to fall outside of the guidelines for expected number of visits. These need to be discussed in the evaluation part of the note. Team meetings, clinical instructors, mentors, other staff members, and class notes can serve as references for setting Expected Outcomes while gaining experience. Be patient with yourself as you learn to set realistic time frames.

Revision

Occasionally, Expected Outcomes may require revision if (1) the patient's condition changes and does not allow progression to the functional level originally set, (2) the patient's condition changes and allows progression beyond the functional level originally set, or (3) the time span set is no longer appropriate and should be revised.

Relationship to the Examination, Evaluation, Diagnosis, and Prognosis

Once the examination of a patient is complete, the therapist documents the patient's functional deficits and impairments and discusses their relationship in the evaluation part of the note, places them in a practice pattern and possibly another diagnostic category, and discusses the patient's overall prognosis. Then the therapist writes the Expected Outcomes based on the functional deficits listed, the evaluation, the diagnosis, and the prognosis written.

To use a previous example, the following are excerpts from an initial note that you wrote (first written in Patient/Client Management Note format and then in the SOAP Note format; the Patient/Client Management format will be used for this example):

example

History: <u>Demographics:</u> Pt. is a 65 y.o. ♂ c̄ a dx of DJD Ⓡ hip c̄ a THA on [date]. Physician is Dr. Sienn. Pt. is Ⓡ-hand dominant. <u>Current Condition:</u> c/o Ⓡ hip pain in area of sutures of the following intensities: 7 when moving, 3 when sitting, 2 when lying still (0 = no pain, 10 = worst possible pain). Does not recall precautions for Pts. c̄ THA. PTA pain was constant & intensity was 9 or 10. <u>Pt. goals:</u> Pt. wants to eventually return to gardening & yard work activities. <u>Prior Level of Function:</u> Immediately PTA, PT. amb. s̄ assist. device. PTA attempted amb. for exercise daily; was only able to amb. 1 block PTA. Two yrs. ago Pt. was able to amb. 1 mi. or more. <u>Social Hx:</u> Lives c̄ his wife in his own home. Plans to return home c̄ his wife p̄ D/C. <u>Employment:</u> Pt. is retired. <u>Living Environment:</u> Has 1 step to enter home c̄ railing on Ⓡ ascending. Owns a 3-in-1 commode, a walker, & a cane. <u>General Health Status:</u> Pt. rates general health as good; no major life changes in past yr. <u>Social/Health Habits:</u> Does not smoke; only occasionally drinks ETOH. <u>Family Hx:</u> Pt.'s father died of MI at age 78. Pt.'s mother died of breast CA at age 72. Pt. has no siblings. <u>Medical/ Surgical Hx:</u> Hx of htn. Hx of hospitalization for Ⓛ THA on 1/10/2007. <u>Functional Status/ Activity Level:</u> Hobby is gardening. Gardens outside of the church. Does volunteer ushering at church. <u>Medications:</u> Takes [antihypertensive medication]. ─────────────

─────────────────────────────

─────────────

Systems Review: <u>Cardiovascular/pulmonary:</u> not impaired. HR 80 bpm. Resp. rate 14 breaths/ min. BP 130/85. Edema: none noted. <u>Integumentary:</u> impaired. Disruption: staples Ⓡ hip. Skin color WNL. Skin texture not tested this date. <u>Musculoskeletal:</u> Gross symmetry not impaired. Gross ROM & strength impaired Ⓡ hip & knee. Ht: 6 ft. 0 in. Wt: 185 lbs. <u>Neuromuscular:</u> Gait impaired. Locomotion: impaired transfers & bed mobility. Balance impaired in standing; uses walker. Not impaired in sitting. Motor function not impaired. <u>Communication</u> not impaired.

<u>Cognition</u>: oriented ×3; not impaired. <u>Learning barriers</u>: cannot read s̄ glasses. <u>Education needs</u>: home exercise program, precautions for Pts c̄ THA, progression of recovery process, use of walker, ADLs including transfers. <u>Learning style</u>: prefers demonstration ā trying an activity; visual learner.

Tests & Measures: <u>Amb</u>: Stood B/S c̄ walker 10% PWB Ⓡ LE c̄ mod. assist. of 1 for 1 minute ×2. <u>Transfers</u>: Supine ↔ sit c min. assist of 1. Sit ↔ stand & w/c ↔ mat pivot c̄ mod. assist. of 1. Toilet transfers not tested this date. Ⓡ LE: Strength grossly 1/5 in hip & knee musculature; ankle dorsiflexion 4+/5; ankle plantar flexion at least 2/5 but not tested further due to 10% PWB status. PROM: 0–20° hip flexion, 0–10° hip abduction, 0° hip extension; adduction, medial & lateral rotation of hip not tested due to hip precautions & recent surgery. Knee flexion: 0–70°. AROM Ⓡ ankle WNL. Incision Ⓡ hip 10 cm long over greater trochanter; staples intact. UE & Ⓛ LE: AROM WNL & strength 4+/5 throughout bilat. UEs & Ⓛ LE. Group muscle testing performed UEs; individual muscle testing performed LEs.

Evaluation: Indep. amb. c̄ a walker is necessary for Pt. to return to home. Impairments of ↓ ROM & strength Ⓡ LE are associated with dependent amb. on this date.

Diagnosis: Practice Pattern Musculoskeletal H: Impaired Joint Mobility, Motor Function, Muscle Performance & ROM Associated c̄ Joint Arthroplasty.

Prognosis: Pt. has good rehab. potential. His level of function was good PTA & he has a great desire to return to a healthy, active lifestyle in the community. Should be able to return home c̄ his wife indep. in amb. & a home exercise program to cont. to ↑ Ⓡ LE strength & ROM c̄ 2-3 days of therapy BID.

The expected outcomes (what will be achieved by the time the patient is discharged from the hospital in 3 days) are as follows:

1. Indep. transfers on/off toilet, supine ↔ sit, sit ↔ stand, chair ↔ bed, so Pt. is safe for ADL at home within 3 days. (This addresses the functional deficit concerning transfers.)

2. Indep. walker amb. FWB **R** LE for at least 150 ft. ×2 on level surfaces & on 1 step within 3 days so Pt. can function indep in amb. at home. (This addresses the functional deficit concerning ambulation.)

Setting Priorities

Expected Outcomes are listed in order of priority. Often, the most important or more vital functional activity is listed first. In the previous example, transfers were listed first because a patient can perform safe transfers and must do so whether or not the patient is independent in ambulation. For the purposes of this workbook, you are not expected to set expected outcome priorities. You will be guided on what the outcomes should be and how to set priorities. Often, the outcomes on the worksheets will be given to you in order of priority.

Relationship to Anticipated Goals

Anticipated Goals are written as steps along the way to achieving expected outcomes.

example

Expected Outcome
Indep. amb. c̄ a walker FWB Ⓡ LE for at least 150 ft. ×2 on level surfaces & on 1 step elevation within 1 mo. to allow Pt. to amb. around her house.

Anticipated Goal
Pt. will amb. 30 ft. ×2 in parallel bars 10% PWB Ⓡ LE within 3 days c̄ mod. +1 assist. to progress Pt. toward amb. household distances.

Anticipated Goal (Later in the Patient's Progress)
Pt. will amb. c̄ a walker 60 ft. ×2 10% PWB Ⓡ LE within 1 wk. c̄ min. +1 assist. to progress Pt. toward amb. household distances.

Anticipated Goals also address impairments that affect the patient's ability to perform functional activities, such as range of motion and strength associated with decreased function in ambulation and transfers for patients who have had a total joint arthroplasty.

As you can see in the following example, the Anticipated Goals include educational goals and goals that address the impairments. Notice that the first anticipated goal in the example specifically tied the impairment with the functional activity involved. To summarize, Anticipated Goals can address issues of function, impairments, and education for the patient that are implied or stated in the Expected Outcomes.

example

(Using the previous case)

Expected Outcome

1. Indep. transfers on/off toilet, supine↔sit, sit↔stand, chair↔bed, so Pt. is safe for ADL at home within 3 days. (This covers the functional deficit concerning transfers.)

Anticipated Goals

1. Pt. will ↑ Ⓡ hip flexion AROM to 0–80° within 3 days to assist. c̄ indep. transfers so Pt. can progress to safe ADLs for home.
2. Pt. will perform home exercise program to ↑ Ⓡ hip & knee AROM & strength indep. within 3 days to assist. c̄ indep. transfers so Pt. can progress to safe ADLs for home.
3. Pt. will ↑ strength Ⓡ hip abduction and flexion to at least 3/5 within 3 days to assist. c̄ indep. transfers and amb. so Pt. can progress to safe ADLs & amb. for home.

A Word About Discharge Summaries

When writing a discharge summary, list the expected outcomes and most recent anticipated goals, indicating which expected outcomes and anticipated goals have been achieved and which have not been achieved. This is particularly important for the Expected Outcomes section because Expected Outcomes, by definition, list the functional status the patient is to achieve by discharge from PT for the patient's current condition. If the patient has not achieved expected outcomes, the patient should be referred for therapy in another type of setting (e.g., outpatient or home health when the patient is discharged from acute care). If the outcomes have not been achieved and therapy in another setting is not recommended, or the patient is not referred for therapy in another type of setting, a reason for the patient not achieving the outcomes should be listed.

A Word About Progress Notes

When writing a progress note, Expected Outcomes are usually not addressed unless they are achieved or need to be revised.

Summary and Objective

Outcomes state the long-term plans for the patient in therapy. It is important that they are structured and clearly defined. They are based on the examination, evaluation, diagnosis, and prognosis. Expected Outcomes require the clinical judgment of the therapist to set the parameters of each goal. Expected Outcomes are functional in nature, whereas Anticipated Goals address both function and impairments.

The worksheets that follow will assist you in setting Expected Outcomes and give you practice in writing outcomes. They will also let you analyze several outcomes, letting you see how each outcome is structured. After you review the previous material, complete the worksheets, and compare your work to the answers in Appendix A, you should be able to write an Expected Outcome correctly when given the parameters, recognize when an Expected Outcome is incomplete, and state the components missing from an incomplete Expected Outcome.

References

1. American Physical Therapy Association: Guide to Physical Therapist Practice, ed. 2, and CD-ROM. American Physical Therapy Association, Alexandria, VA, 2003.
2. American Physical Therapy Association: Defensible Documentation for Patient/Client Management. Accessed at http://www.apta.org/AM/Template.cfm?Section= Documentation4&Template=/MembersOnly. cfm&ContentID=37776 on March 9, 2007.
3. Teaching Improvement Project Systems for Health Care Educators: Instructional Objectives. Center for Learning Resources, College of Allied Health Professions, University of Kentucky, Lexington, KY.

Writing Expected Outcomes (Long-Term Goals):

> ■ **PART I.** In each of the following examples, identify the (A) audience, (B) behavior, (C) condition, and (D) degree.

1. Indep. w/c management & propulsion for approx. 50 ft. ×10 at home within 1 mo. to allow Pt. to function at home.

   A. _____

   B. _____

   C. _____

   D. _____

   _____

   _____

   _____

2. Within 2 wks. Pt. will demonstrate indep. amb. c̄ prosthesis s̄ assist. device on at least 14 stairs & for at least ¹/₂ mi. on even & uneven surfaces to assure Pt.'s ability to amb. in & out of his home & around his yard.

   A. _____

   B. _____

   C. _____

   D. _____

   _____

   _____

   _____

3. Pt. will demonstrate good body mechanics while lifting up to 50 lbs. in order to allow Pt. to return to work fully functional at performing his job within 4 wks. of Rx.

   A. _____

   B. _____

   C. _____

   D. _____

   _____

   _____

   _____

4. Pt. will demonstrate indep. segmental rolling p̄ 6 mo. of Rx in order to make Pt. more functional as she sleeps & plays.

A. _____

B. _____

C. _____

D. _____

_____

_____

_____

PART II. Given the following components of an expected outcome, write them into an expected outcome.

1. A. Pt.
   B. will amb. (will demonstrate amb.)
   C. c̄ crutches,
      on level surfaces & 1 step elevation,
      NWB Ⓛ LE
   D. indep. (observable)
      p̄ 2 days (time span)
      40 ft. ×3 (measurable)
      to allow Pt. to get around her house for ADL (functional)

   Expected Outcome: _____

   _____

   _____

2. A. Pt.
   B. will demonstrate care & wrapping of her residual limb
   C. c̄ elastic wrap
   D. indep. (observable)
      applying even pressure (observable)
      100% of the time (measurable)
      to prepare for training in amb. c̄ a prosthesis (functional)
      within 3 days (time span)

   Expected Outcome: _____

   _____

   _____

3. A. Pt.
   B. will be able to lift a box
   C. from an overhead cupboard to place it on a table
   D. using bilat. UEs equally (observable)
      within 2 mo. (time span)
      in order to enable Pt.'s ability to reach items on the shelves in her kitchen & closets at home during ADL (functional)
      box will weigh 5 lbs. (measurable)

   Expected Outcome: _____

   _____

   _____

4. A. Pt.
   B. will amb.
   C. in her home
      s̄ an assist. device
   D. for 50 ft. ×4 (measurable)
      using pursed lip breathing pattern (observable)
      to enable her to cook & perform ADLs (functional)
      p̄ 4 wks. of Rx.

Expected Outcome: _____

_____

_____

■ PART III. Write the appropriate Expected Outcomes as described below.

EVALUATION: Pt.'s inability to lift pots & pans in her kitchen & inability to reach items in her overhead kitchen cabinets is caused by ↓ Ⓡ elbow flexion & extension AROM & ↓ Ⓡ biceps & triceps strength. This inability is preventing Pt. from being able to indep. function in her kitchen.

DIAGNOSIS: Practice Pattern Musculoskeletal G: Impaired Joint Mobility, Muscle Performance, & ROM Associated c̄ Fx.

PROGNOSIS: Pt. has good rehab. potential. Should improve quickly, within 10 visits, c̄ follow up of Pt. performing home exercise program between therapy visits.

Use the instructions below to formulate an Expected Outcome for each functional deficit mentioned.

1. The Pt. is unable to lift pots and pans in her kitchen. You judge that by D/C, the Pt. should be able to lift pots and pans up to 20 pounds and function indep. in her kitchen.

Expected Outcome: _____

_____

_____

_____

2. The Pt. is unable to reach items in her overhead kitchen cabinets. You judge that by D/C the Pt. should be able to reach items in overhead cabinets up to 5 ft. 10 in. so that she can function indep. in her kitchen.

Expected Outcome: _____

_____

_____

_____

Answers to "Writing Expected Outcomes: Worksheet 1" are provided in Appendix A.

Writing Expected Outcomes (Long-Term Goals)

> ■ **PART I.** In each of the following examples, identify the (A) audience, (B) behavior, (C) condition, and (D) degree.

1. Indep. amb. c̄ straight cane for 150 ft. ×2 on level surfaces & on at least 5 stairs within 1 wk. so Pt.'s level of indep. at home ↑.

   A. _____

   B. _____

   C. _____

   D. _____

   _____

   _____

   _____

2. Pt.'s wife will indep. transfer Pt. w/c↔supine in bed & w/c↔toilet giving min. +1 assist. to Pt. p̄ 2 wks. of Rx & 5 sessions of family teaching so wife can care for Pt. at home.

   A. _____

   B. _____

   C. _____

   D. _____

   _____

   _____

   _____

3. Indep. transfers w/c ↔ floor within 3 mo. of Rx so Pt. can safely play on the floor c̄ her siblings.

   A. _____

   B. _____

   C. _____

   D. _____

   _____

   _____

   _____

> **PART II.** Given the following components of an expected outcome, write them into the expected outcome.

1. A. Pt.
   B. will sit
   C. on the edge of a mat or chair
   D. s̄ falling (observable)
      for at least 10 min. (measurable)
      p̄ 2 mo. of Rx (time span)
      to allow Pt. to more safely function at school (function)

   Expected Outcome: _____

   _____

   _____

   _____

2. A. Pt.
   B. will transfer supine↔sit, sit↔stand, on/off toilet
   C. toilet c̄ raised toilet seat & some surface (mat or bed) on which to lie are necessary
   D. independent (observable)
      p̄ 2 wks. of Rx (time span)
      in order for Pt. to function indep. at home (function)

   Expected Outcome: _____

   _____

   _____

   _____

3. A. Pt.
   B. will propel w/c
   C. on level surfaces including tiled and carpeted surfaces
   D. independently (observable)
      after one month of therapy (time span)
      to increase Pt.'s independence at home (functional)

   Expected Outcome: _____

   _____

   _____

   _____

> **PART III.** Write the Expected Outcomes as described below.

Case: You have just completed writing the Examination, Diagnosis, and Prognosis portions of a note.

EVALUATION: Pt.'s gait deviations are caused by ↓ ROM Ⓛ knee & ↓ strength Ⓛ quadriceps. Pt. is not indep. & safe in amb. c̄ walker & transfers so Pt. cannot return to home at this time because he lives alone.

DIAGNOSIS: Practice Pattern Musculoskeletal H: Impaired Joint Mobility, Motor Function, Muscle Performance, & ROM Associated c̄ Joint Arthroplasty.

PROGNOSIS: Pt. has good rehab. potential & should be able to return to home. Residual deficits in Ⓡ LE from stroke 2 yrs. ago may lengthen rehab. time. Anticipate 2 wk. stay on SNF Unit to prepare Pt. to be fully functional & safe at home.

Use the following instructions to formulate an expected outcome for each functional deficit mentioned.

Expected Outcomes:

1. The patient is not safe in ambulation. You believe patient will ambulate with a walker on level surfaces and 3 stairs with a handrail full weight bearing as tolerated by discharge in 2 weeks so he can get around his home independently.

   Expected Outcome: _____

   _____

   _____

   _____

2. The patient is unable to transfer independently. You judge that by discharge the patient should be able to transfer bed to/from chair, sit to/from stand, on/off the toilet independently to allow the patient to function at home alone.

   Expected Outcome: _____

   _____

   _____

   _____

Answers to "Writing Expected Outcomes: Worksheet 2" are provided in Appendix A.

15 | Writing Anticipated Goals (Short-Term Goals)

Anticipated Goals are part of the Plan of Care portion of the note. They are the interim steps along the way to achieving Expected Outcomes (the final product of therapeutic intervention). Once the Expected Outcomes of therapy have been determined, the Anticipated Goals are then set. The specific regimen of interventions is designed to achieve the Anticipated Goals.

Reasons for Writing Goals

Anticipated Goals are written for several reasons. These reasons include:

1) to direct interventions to the specific needs and problems of the patients,
2) to set priorities in interventions and measure the effectiveness of interventions,
3) to assist with cost-effectiveness (for purposes of third-party payment), and
4) to communicate therapy goals to other health care professionals.

Anticipated Goals help to guide the immediate Intervention Plan. Periodically reviewing and resetting Anticipated Goals help the therapist and patient realize the progress that the patient has made.

The Structure of Anticipated Goals

Like Expected Outcomes, Anticipated Goals are objectives, and they need to contain the following elements that a good objective contains:

A. Audience
B. Behavior
C. Condition
D. Degree

A brief review of the definitions of the elements of a goal with examples from Anticipated Goals follows.

Audience

Almost always, the audience is the patient. However, the audience *can* be a family member, as in "Pt.'s wife will wrap Pt.'s residual limb c̄ 3 in. elastic wrap c̄ verbal cues only p̄ 4 visits to prepare Pt. for amb. training c̄ a prosthesis." Often the audience is implied in goal writing,

and it is not necessary to say, "Pt. will demonstrate ..." or "Pt. will ..."

Behavior

This is always indicated by a verb followed by the object of the behavior. Good examples are "↑ Ⓡ knee AROM ...," "↓ dependence in dressing," and "improve gait pattern ..." The object of the behavior must be something that can be *measured* or *described accurately* so that an increase or improvement can be documented at a later date.

Condition

Condition includes the circumstances under which the behavior must be done. Examples are "↓ dependence in *walker* amb. to min + 1 assist. within 1 wk.," "indep. amb. s̄ *assistive device on level surfaces* for 10 ft. ×2 within 1 wk."

Sometimes the circumstances under which the behavior must be done are implied. If "Normal pain-free Ⓡ LE AROM & strength" is set as an outcome, it is implied that you must have a goniometer available and strength will be measured via manual muscle testing.

Degree

Degree includes the minimal number, the percentage or proportion, any limitation or departure from a fixed standard, or any distinguishing features of successful performance. It also includes standards such as the time span after which the therapist anticipates that the goal will be achieved.

When writing goals, the degree of performance must be *realistic, measurable,* or *observable;* must name a specific *time span;* and should *tie into functional activities* listed in the outcomes.

Consider the example of a goal given previously: "Pt.'s wife will wrap Pt.'s residual limb c̄ 3-in. elastic wrap c̄ *verbal cues only* (measurable) p̄ *4 visits* (time span) *to prepare Pt. for training in amb. c̄ a prosthesis* (functional terms)."

Review this goal and analyze its parts: "Pt.'s wife will wrap Pt.'s residual limb c̄ 3-in. elastic wrap c̄ verbal cues only p̄ 4 visits to prepare Pt. for prosthetic training."

A. Pt.'s wife
B. will wrap Pt.'s residual limb

C. c̄ 3-in. elastic wrap
D. c̄ verbal cues only (observable) c̄ 4 visits (time span) to prepare Pt. for amb. training c̄ prosthesis (functional)

Another example follows: "↑ AROM Ⓡ knee flexion to 5–55° within 3 days to improve transfers & gait."

A. Pt. (implied)
B. will ↑ Ⓡ knee flexion AROM
C. no conditions given (assumed: goniometer will be used)
D. 5–55° (measurable) within 3 days (time span) to improve Pt.'s transfers & gait (functional)

Functional Terms

Therapists at some facilities do not add the final phrase to the goal to put it in functional terms. The advantage of using the final phrase in the previous examples is to notify third-party payors and other health professionals of the functional reasons for the goal. Among rehabilitation professionals, it is generally known that the patient will not be very functional in transfers and ambulation with a knee with very little AROM; however, this is not always so clear to others. The goal of wrapping the residual limb is not always clear to all health care professionals working with the patient and certainly could confuse third-party payors if this is one of the patient's goals. Including functional terms is the preferred method for writing all goals.

If an explanation of a goal is needed and stating the goal in functional terms is not adequate to explain the reasons for setting the goal, it should be explained further under the Evaluation part of the note.

Some therapists assume that if the Expected Outcomes are functional and the Anticipated Goals correspond well with the Expected Outcomes, then the functional reasons for the Anticipated Goals are obvious. However, the relationship between the Expected Outcomes and Anticipated Goals is not as obvious as therapists may assume. Other therapists always use function and only state Anticipated Goals in functional terms. This varies from facility to facility. You will adapt your style of writing Anticipated Goals as you adapt to various clinical settings.

Clarity

Poorly written Anticipated Goals do not clearly communicate the purpose of therapy for the patient. If certain components of a well-written goal are not included (such as time span, functional terms, or measurable terms), the purpose of interventions may be very unclear. The lack of clarity will be especially confusing to third-party payors and health care professionals who are not familiar with therapy interventions and their purposes. At times, the goal must be related to patient function for the purpose of communicating clearly to those reading the patient care note.

Time Span

Anticipated Goals are patient objectives that have a time span for their achievement. The most common time frame for Anticipated Goals is a week. However, the time frame can be a few days or longer than a week, depending on the patient's diagnosis and general condition. For example, a patient with a brain injury may take 3 to 4 months for rehabilitation at times, so Anticipated Goals can be set weekly or for a 2-week period. Other patients in some pediatric settings may have Expected Outcomes set for 1 year and Anticipated Goals may be set for 1 to 3 months.

Setting the Time Span.   Setting a specific time span after which a goal will be achieved is difficult, especially for new practitioners, because it takes clinical experience to know how quickly a patient will progress. At times, even experienced clinicians have difficulty predicting how quickly a patient will progress. Generally, a clinician can consider when a note on a particular patient must be written again and what the therapist anticipates the patient's status will be at that time. If the patient's status will change by the time a note is due to be written, the time span can be set to correspond with the date the note is due. If achieving a goal will take longer, choose a longer time span. If it will take less time, set a shorter time span. Remember, Anticipated Goals can always be revised if the time span set is not correct. Clinical instructors, peers, *The Guide to Physical Therapist Practice*,[1] and class notes can serve as references for setting realistic time spans.

At times, Anticipated Goals are not necessary because of an anticipated extremely short patient length of stay. For example, if the patient is only to be seen by a therapist one or two times, the Expected Outcomes may be adequate and Anticipated Goals are not needed. If the Expected Outcomes imply or require an improvement at the impairment level, Anticipated Goals may be set.

Revision

Anticipated Goals must be revised periodically. An anticipated goal should be revised if (1) the period mentioned in the goal has passed, or (2) the patient has achieved the goals set. Consider a previous example: "↓ dependence in walker amb. to min. +1 assist. for 10 ft. ×2 within 1 wk. to facilitate indep. walker amb. at home."

Assume 3 days have passed and the patient required minimal of 1 assistance and is progressing. The goal is reset to read: "↓ dependence in walker amb. to contact guard assist. for 60 ft. ×4 within 1 wk. to facilitate amb. functional distances needed for home."

Another week passes and the patient's rate of progress has decreased. The therapist now comments on lack of progress and resets the anticipated goal: "Goal to ↓ amb. dependence not yet achieved due to ... (It is good to give a reason if there is one.) Will ↓ dependence in amb. c̄ walker to contact guard assist. for 60 ft. ×4 within 1 more wk. of Rx."

Relationship to Expected Outcomes

Anticipated Goals are written as steps along the way to achieving Expected Outcomes.

> **example**
>
> **Expected Outcome**
> Indep. amb. c̄ a walker FWB Ⓡ LE for at least 150 ft. ×2 on level surfaces & on 1 step elevation within 3 wks. to allow Pt. to amb. around her house.
>
> **Anticipated Goal**
> Pt. will amb. 5 ft. ×2 at B/S c̄ a walker 10% PWB Ⓡ LE within 1 wk. c̄ mod. +1 assist. to progress Pt. toward amb. at home.
>
> **Anticipated Goal (Later on in the Patient's Progress)**
> Pt. will amb. c̄ a walker on the nursing floor 10% PWB Ⓡ LE for 50 ft. ×2, including turns within 2 wks. c̄ min. +1 assist to progress Pt. toward amb. at home.

Anticipated Goals also address impairments that affect the patient's ability to perform functional activities, such as range of motion and strength affecting ambulation and transfers for patients who have had a total joint arthroplasty.

Anticipated Goals include educational goals and goals that address the impairments. Notice that the first anticipated goal in the example specifically tied the impairment with the functional activity involved. In summary, Anticipated Goals can address issues of function, impairments, and education for the patient that are implied or stated in the Expected Outcomes.

> **example**
>
> Using the previous case:
>
> **Expected Outcome (one of several listed in the Pt. documentation)**
> 1. Indep. transfers on/off toilet, supine↔sit, sit↔stand, chair↔bed, so Pt. is safe for ADL at home within 3 days. (This covers the functional deficit concerning transfers.)
>
> **Anticipated Goals**
> 1. Pt. will ↑ Ⓡ hip flexion AROM to 0–85° within 1 wk. to assist. c̄ indep. transfers & amb.
> 2. Pt. will perform exercise program in her room to ↑ Ⓡ hip & knee AROM & strength indep. within 1 wk. to assist. c̄ indep. transfers & amb.
> 3. Pt. will ↑ strength Ⓡ hip abduction & flexion to at least 3/5 within 1 wk. to assist. c̄ indep. transfers & amb.

Setting Priorities

Priorities are set for Anticipated Goals by looking at the priorities set for the Expected Outcomes. If the Expected Outcomes are listed in order of priority and the Anticipated Goals are set to meet the Expected Outcomes, the Anticipated Goals already have a priority order. If there is more than one anticipated goal for a particular expected outcome, as in the previous example, the Anticipated Goals for that outcome are listed with the most functional goal (such as ambulation or transfers) listed first. Anticipated Goals that address impairments (such as range of motion or strength) usually follow more functional Anticipated Goals.

For the purposes of this workbook, you are not expected to set goal priorities. You will be guided in setting the goals and in setting goal priorities if the priorities are different from those of the Expected Outcomes or if there are two or more Anticipated Goals that correspond to one expected outcome.

Relationship to the Intervention Plan

When Anticipated Goals are set, the therapist (with the patient's input) determines the interventions for the next few days. When an intervention plan is set, an intervention to work toward *each* of the Anticipated Goals must be included.

> **example**
>
> **Expected Outcomes (to be achieved within 2 wks.)**
> 1. indep. walker amb. on level surfaces FWB for 70 ft. ×2, including turns & obstacles, & on 1 step. so Pt. can get in & out of her home & amb. within her home safely.
> 2. indep. transfers chair↔bed, sit↔stand, on/off toilet so Pt. can function indep. & safely at home.
>
> **Anticipated Goals (To be achieved within 1 wk.)**
> 1. Pt. will amb. c̄ walker 50% PWB Ⓡ LE for ~20 ft. ×2 to progress toward amb. at home (*from first expected outcome*).
> 2. Pt. will transfer bed↔chair & sit↔stand c̄ min. assist. of 1 to progress toward transfers at home (*from second expected outcome*).

3. Pt. will ↑ ®quadriceps strength to at least 2/5 to ↑ indep. in amb. & transfers (*from first and second Expected Outcomes*).
4. Pt. will indep. demonstrate exercises that he is to perform in the hopsital room that ↑ ® LE strength to progress Pt. toward indep. amb. & transfers (*from first and second Expected Outcomes*).

Intervention Plan

<u>BID at B/S:</u> Amb. training c̄ a walker, beginning c̄ 50% PWB & progressing to wt. bearing & distance as tolerated (*from first anticipated goal*). Transfer training, beginning c̄ bed↔chair & sit↔stand & progressing to on/off toilet (*from second anticipated goal—placed second in priority because it is functional*). Pt will be given written & verbal instruction in exercise program to ↑ ® LE strength to be performed in the hospital room between Rx sessions (attached) (*from fourth anticipated goal*). AAROM progressing to AROM exercises ® knee, emphasizing quadriceps function (*from third anticipated goal*).

Sometimes an intervention works toward more than one anticipated goal at a time, as demonstrated in the previous example. Further explanation of the relationship of the intervention plan to the Anticipated Goals is discussed in Chapter 16.

Anticipated Goals in Progress Notes

When writing a progress note, the therapist refers to the Anticipated Goals previously set and sets new Anticipated Goals if the previous Anticipated Goals have been achieved. If an anticipated goal previously set has not yet been achieved, the therapist comments on the reason it has not yet been achieved. Then the therapist either resets the goal to make it more reasonable or restates the goal as a goal to be achieved by the next progress note to be written.

example

Anticipated Goals
Goal #4 of [date] for amb. c̄ walker 10% PWB ® LE for 20 ft. ×2 c̄ mod. +1 assist. not yet achieved due to ↓ in Pt.'s medical status; Pt. will be able to achieve this goal c̄ 1 more wk. of PT.

example

Anticipated Goals
All achieved. Will work directly toward Expected Outcomes set on [date].

Anticipated Goals in Discharge Notes

When writing a discharge summary, the therapist may comment on the most recently set Anticipated Goals as to whether or not they were achieved and why. However, in a discharge summary, the emphasis should be on the Expected Outcomes and why they were or were not achieved or the services still needed to assist the patient in achieving those outcomes.

Summary and Objective

Setting Anticipated Goals is the second step in the Plan of Care part of the note. Anticipated Goals are based on the Expected Outcomes and direct the immediate course of the Intervention Plan. The period covered by Anticipated Goals is briefer than that for Expected Outcomes. Revision of Anticipated Goals is done on a regular basis and generally indicates that the patient is making progress. Setting Anticipated Goals involves professional judgment.

The worksheets that follow will assist you in setting Anticipated Goals and will give you practice in writing the goals. They will also let you analyze several goals, allowing you to see how each goal is structured. After reviewing the previous material, completing the worksheets, and comparing your work to the answers in Appendix A, you should be able to write an Anticipated Goal correctly when given the parameters of the goal, recognize when a goal is incomplete, and state the components missing from an incomplete Anticipated Goal.

References

1. American Physical Therapy Association: Guide to Physical Therapist Practice, ed. 2, and CD-ROM. American Physical Therapy Association, Alexandria, VA, 2003.
2. American Physical Therapy Association: Defensible Documentation for Patient/Client Management. Accessed at http://www.apta.org/AM/Template.cfm?Section= Documentation4&Template=/MembersOnly. cfm&ContentID=37776 on March 9, 2007.
3. Teaching Improvement Project Systems for Health Care Educators: Instructional Objectives. Center for Learning Resources, College of Allied Health Professions, University of Kentucky, Lexington, KY.

Writing Anticipated Goals (Short-Term Goals)

> ■ **PART I.** In each of the following examples, identify the audience (A), behavior (B), condition (C), and degree (D).

1. ANTICIPATED GOAL: ↑ Ⓡ shoulder flexion AROM to 0–90° within 6 Rx sessions to work toward Pt. reaching her overhead kitchen cupboards.

   A. _____

   B. _____

   C. _____

   D. _____

   _____

   _____

   _____

2. ANTICIPATED GOAL: Pt. will grasp object in midline 3 out of 4 times within 3 mo. in order to ↑ Pt's functional use of his UEs during ADLs.

   A. _____

   B. _____

   C. _____

   D. _____

   _____

   _____

   _____

3. ANTICIPATED GOAL: Pt. will demonstrate good body mechanics by correct performance of at least 90% of tasks in obstacle course p̄ 3 Rx sessions to prevent further Pt. injury at work.

   A. _____

   B. _____

   C. _____

   D. _____

   _____

   _____

   _____

> **PART II.** Given the following components of a goal, write them into an anticipated goal.

1. A. Pt.
   B. will amb.
   C. using a walker on level surfaces only NWB 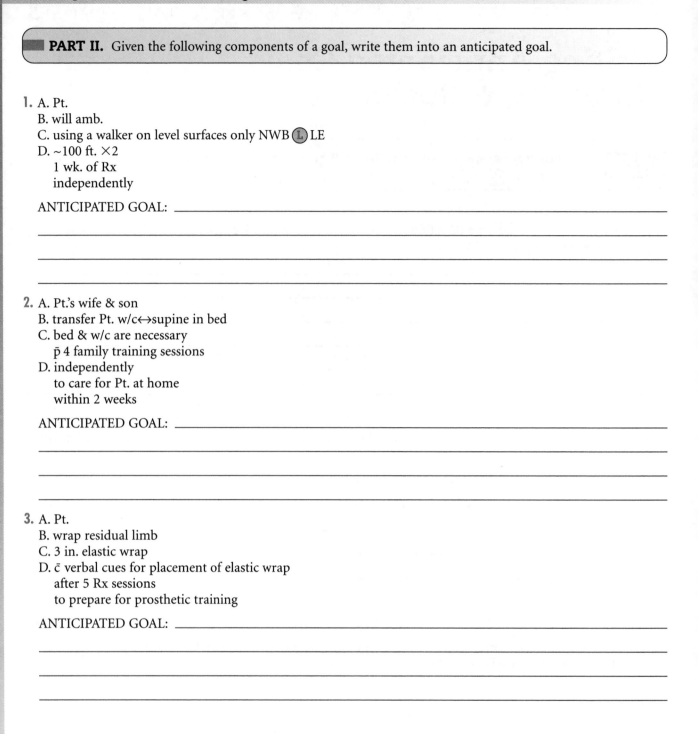Ⓛ LE
   D. ~100 ft. ×2
      1 wk. of Rx
      independently

   ANTICIPATED GOAL: _____

   _____

   _____

   _____

2. A. Pt.'s wife & son
   B. transfer Pt. w/c↔supine in bed
   C. bed & w/c are necessary
      p̄ 4 family training sessions
   D. independently
      to care for Pt. at home
      within 2 weeks

   ANTICIPATED GOAL: _____

   _____

   _____

   _____

3. A. Pt.
   B. wrap residual limb
   C. 3 in. elastic wrap
   D. c̄ verbal cues for placement of elastic wrap
      after 5 Rx sessions
      to prepare for prosthetic training

   ANTICIPATED GOAL: _____

   _____

   _____

   _____

> ■ **PART III.** In each of the following cases, write the appropriate anticipated goal.

Case 1

TESTS & MEASURES: Requires verbal cues & mod + 1 assist. to don/doff prosthesis Ⓡ LE
EVALUATION: Functional limitations: dependent in donning/doffing prosthesis Ⓡ LE, a skill needed for indep. amb.
c̄ prosthesis Ⓡ LE.
DIAGNOSIS & PROGNOSIS: . . .
EXPECTED OUTCOME: Indep. donning/doffing prosthesis in 1 wk. to allow Pt. to come to standing.

ANTICIPATED GOAL: _____

_____

_____

_____

You judge that 1 week from now only contact guard assistance of one person and no verbal cues will be needed for the patient to don and doff his prosthesis. The functional purpose of this is to assist with sit to stand transfers. Write the anticipated goal above.

Case 2

MEDICAL DX: stroke c̄ Ⓛ sided weakness.
TESTS & MEASURES: Amb: Stands in parallel bars c̄ mod +1 assist. & verbal cues for wt. shift. Wt. shift onto
Ⓛ LE is poor; Pt. bears only 10 lbs. of wt. on Ⓛ LE. ↓ wt. shift onto Ⓛ LE is ↑ Pt.'s dependence in amb.
EVALUATION: Functional limitation: dependent ambulation c̄ ↓ wt. shift onto Ⓛ LE.
DIAGNOSIS & PROGNOSIS: ...
EXPECTED OUTCOME: Indep. amb. c̄ straight cane for unlimited distances c̄ normal gait pattern, including normal wt. shift onto Ⓛ LE p̄ 4 wks. of therapy.

ANTICIPATED GOAL: _____

_____

_____

_____

You judge that in 1 week minimal assistance of one person and verbal cues will be needed for the patient to be able to ambulate with a straight cane for 10 feet with at least half of his body weight shifted onto his left leg.

Case 3

MEDICAL DX: L4 herniated disc. Lumbar laminectomy performed on [date].
TESTS & MEASURES: <u>Trunk</u>: Can tolerate lying prone for 5 min. Cannot tolerate further trunk extension.
EVALUATION: Pt. is non-functional in lying prone & has the impairment of pain while lying prone.
EXPECTED OUTCOME: Pt. will be able to perform all ADLs s̄ pain p̄ 8 Rx.

ANTICIPATED GOAL: _____

_____

_____

_____

You judge that after 2 Rx sessions the patient will be pain free in the prone-on elbow position for 5 minutes. This will progress the patient toward independence in ADLs.

> **PART IV.** State which components each of the following Anticipated Goals are missing.

1. ANTICIPATED GOAL: Pt. will be able to perform sliding board transfers.

Missing components: _____

_____

2. ANTICIPATED GOAL: Pt. will demonstrate the correct position for hip flexor stretching.

Missing components: _____

_____

3. ANTICIPATED GOAL: 10-min. exercise routine s̄ fatigue within 5 wks.

Missing components: _____

_____

Answers to "Writing Anticipated Goals: Worksheet 1" are provided in Appendix A.

Writing Anticipated Goals (Short-Term Goals)

> ■ **PART I.** In each of the following examples, identify the audience (A), behavior (B), condition (C), and degree (D).

1. ANTICIPATED GOAL: p̄ 6 Rx sessions, Pt. will ↑ exercise tolerance as demonstrated by max. ↑ resp. rate of 5 breaths/min. p̄ amb. s̄ device for 150 ft. to ↑ Pt. function in ADLs & IADLs at home.

   A. _____

   B. _____

   C. _____

   D. _____

   _____

   _____

   _____

2. ANTICIPATED GOAL: Pt. will able to long sit propped c̄ a pillow or wedge maintaining good head position 0–45° of neck flexion for 1 min. p̄ 6 wks. of Rx to assist. c̄ Pt. function in the classroom.

   A. _____

   B. _____

   C. _____

   D. _____

   _____

   _____

   _____

3. ANTICIPATED GOAL: Pt. will transfer supine↔sit on a mat using rotation & pushing c̄ his UEs correctly 1 out of 3 attempts within 1 mo. of PT.

   A. _____

   B. _____

   C. _____

   D. _____

   _____

   _____

   _____

> **PART II.**   Given the following components of a goal, write them into an anticipated goal.

1. A. Pt.
   B. hold his head up
   C. while Pt. prone
   D. in midline (*observable*)
      for 15 sec. (*measureable*)
      within 3 mo. of Rx (*time span*)
      to assist Pt.'s ability to learn (*functional terms*)

   ANTICIPATED GOAL: _____

   _____

   _____

   _____

2. A. Pt.
   B. will roll supine↔prone
   C. on a mat
   D. in 6–8 wks.
      indep.
      to assist c̄ Pt.'s indep. at home

   ANTICIPATED GOAL: _____

   _____

   _____

   _____

3. A. Pt.
   B. ambulate stairs with walker
   C. walker & stairs must be available
      50% PWB Ⓡ LE
   D. 5 stairs
      c̄ min. assist. from his wife
      independently
      p̄ 1 week of Rx
      to ↑ Pt. function at home

   ANTICIPATED GOAL: _____

   _____

   _____

   _____

PART III. In each of the following excerpted cases, write the appropriate anticipated goal.

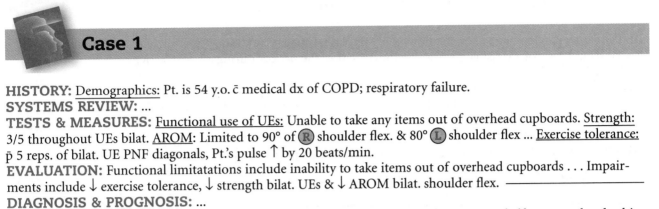

Case 1

HISTORY: Demographics: Pt. is 54 y.o. c̄ medical dx of COPD; respiratory failure.
SYSTEMS REVIEW: ...
TESTS & MEASURES: Functional use of UEs: Unable to take any items out of overhead cupboards. Strength: 3/5 throughout UEs bilat. AROM: Limited to 90° of (R) shoulder flex. & 80° (L) shoulder flex ... Exercise tolerance: p̄ 5 reps. of bilat. UE PNF diagonals, Pt.'s pulse ↑ by 20 beats/min.
EVALUATION: Functional limitatations include inability to take items out of overhead cupboards . . . Impairments include ↓ exercise tolerance, ↓ strength bilat. UEs & ↓ AROM bilat. shoulder flex. ─────────
DIAGNOSIS & PROGNOSIS: ...
EXPECTED OUTCOME: Pt. will be able to retrieve items 5 lbs. in weight from upper shelf over overhead cabinet within 2 wks. to allow Pt. to become more indep. at home. ─────────

ANTICIPATED GOAL: ─────────────────────────

─────────────────────────────────
─────────────────────────────────
─────────────────────────────────
─────────────────────────────────
─────────────────────────────────
─────────────────────────────────
─────────────────────────────────
─────────────────────────────────
─────────────────────────────────
─────────────────────────────────
─────────────────────────────────
─────────────────────────────────
─────────────────────────────────
─────────────────────────────────
─────────────────────────────────

1. You judge that the Pt. will be able to retrieve items 0.5 pounds in weight from the lower shelf of overhead cabinet after 1 week of therapy.

2. You judge that the patient will perform 7 repetitions of each of the 2 PNF patterns for the arms after 1 week of therapy within available AROM to progress the patient toward reaching into her cupboards.

3. You judge that AROM of right shoulder flexion will increase to 100° within 1 week of therapy to progress the patient toward reaching into her cupboards.

4. You judge that AROM of left shoulder flexion will increase to 90° within 1 week of therapy to progress the patient toward reaching into her cupboards.

5. You judge that the strength throughout the bilateral upper extremities will increase to 3+/5 bilat. within available AROM after 1 week of therapy to progress the patient toward reaching into her cupboards.

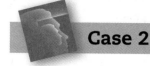

Case 2

HISTORY: <u>Demographics</u>: . . . c̄ a medical dx of whiplash. <u>Current condition</u>: c/o neck pain of an intensity of 9 (0 = no pain, 10 = worst possible pain) c̄ any movement of the neck & during all ADL activities.
SYSTEMS REVIEW: . . .
TESTS & MEASURES: <u>AROM</u>: 0–5° cervical rotation Ⓛ & Ⓡ ; reproduces Pt.'s worst pain.
EVALUATION: Pt. has functional limitations of neck movement during ADL activities. Impairments include pain with all neck movements during ADLs, ↓ AROM in cervical rotation bilat. which reproduces Pt.'s worst pain.
DIAGNOSIS & PROGNOSIS: . . .
EXPECTED OUTCOME: Pt. will be functional in all ADLs s̄ pain in cervical area.

ANTICIPATED GOAL: _____

_____

_____

_____

You judge that the patient will be able to move her head to about 10° of cervical rotation to either side in 2 days to allow the patient to progress toward functional neck movement during ADL activities.

Case 3

HISTORY: <u>Demographics</u>: . . . medical dx is fx Ⓡ tibial plateau c̄ long leg cast applied [date].
SYSTEMS REVIEW: . . .
TESTS & MEASURES: <u>Amb.</u>: c̄ walker 40 ft. ×1 NWB Ⓡ LE c̄ mod. +1 assist.
EVALUATION, DIAGNOSIS, AND PROGNOSIS: . . . .
EXPECTED OUTCOMES: Indep. amb. c̄ crutches for 200 ft. ×4 NWB Ⓡ LE on level surfaces, including turns and obstacles, & stairs within 2 wks. of Rx.

_____

ANTICIPATED GOAL: _____

_____

_____

_____

You judge that the patient will be able to ambulate 40 ft. twice on level surfaces in 1 week with the same weight bearing status and will still require minimal assistance of 1 person to ambulate.

PART IV. State which components of each of the following Anticipated Goals are missing.

1. ANTICIPATED GOALS: ↓ dependence in amb. to min. +1 c̄ walker 40 ft. ×2 NWB Ⓡ LE.

   Missing components: _____

   _____

2. ANTICIPATED GOALS: ↑ Ⓡ shoulder abduction AROM within 3 days.

   Missing components: _____

   _____

3. ANTICIPATED GOALS: ↑ & ↓ stairs c̄ min. + 1 assist.

   Missing components: _____

   _____

Answers to "Writing Anticipated Goals: Worksheet 2" are provided in Appendix A.

16 | Documenting Planned Interventions

*T*he Intervention Plan portion of the note is the final part of the Plan of Care. It contains a plan for the interventions that the patient will receive while in therapy. One or more interventions exist to achieve each of the anticipated goals. Certain information must be included in the intervention plan section of the note, just as certain information is needed for documentation of the examination to be complete.

Information Included Under the Plan

The following information *must be* included in the Intervention Plan section of a note:

- frequency per day or per week that the patient will be seen
- location of the treatment (e.g., at bedside, in the department, in a pool, at home)
- the interventions that the patient will receive in detail (The amount of specificity may depend on the setting. See the following text for more detail on describing interventions. For the purposes of these worksheets, a significant level of detail is expected.)
- if a discharge note, where the patient is going and the number of times the patient was seen in therapy in your setting

The following are also frequently included in the Intervention Plan section:

- planned progression of the interventions
- plans for further examination or re-examination
- plans for discharge
- patient and family education (e.g., home program plans or what was taught to the patient or the patient's family—attach a copy of any home programs [signed and dated, of course] to the note, if possible)
- equipment needs and equipment ordered for or sold to the patient (if a discharge note) and the instruction given to the patient in how to use the equipment
- referral to other services; whether there are plans to consult with the patient's physician regarding further treatment or referral

An example follows:

> **example**
>
> **Intervention Plan:** Will be seen 3×/wk. as an outpatient. Will receive pulsed US to (R) anterior shoulder at 1.5 W/cm² for 5 min. followed

by PROM & AROM exercises to (R) shoulder in saggital, frontal, & transverse planes to ↑ strength & movement of the shoulder. Exercises will be followed c̄ an ice pack to (R) shoulder for 15 min. Pt. will be instructed in home exercise program for (R) shoulder AROM & strengthening (attached).

The Intervention Plan portion of the note intially describes the plan for patient interventions (*what the patient will receive*). This differs from describing the treatment and reaction to treatment mentioned in earlier parts of the note.

The Intervention Plan also describes the specifics of *what was done with the patient that day and/or the patient's reaction to treatment.*

> **example**
>
> **P:** <u>Reaction to Rx:</u> Performed 10 reps each of quad sets & SLR to (L) LE; c̄ 10th repetition of SLR, Pt.'s quadriceps were fatigued & Pt. could no longer perform SLR. <u>Plan:</u> to cont. to see Pt. 1x/wk. to progress home exercise program until Pt. meets outcomes & goals.

Relationship to Anticipated Goals

Once the anticipated goals are set, an Intervention Plan is then set up to achieve each of the anticipated goals. One exercise or intervention may achieve more than one anticipated goal. In fact, it is advantageous and economically sound to establish the intervention program to achieve the goals most efficiently. When setting up an intervention program, each anticipated goal, the patient's allotted time for therapy, the patient's endurance level, and the patient's level of boredom or interest must be considered.

> **example**
>
> **Expected Outcomes**
> 1. Indep. walker amb. on level surfaces FWB for 70 ft. ×2 including obstacles & turns & on 1 step within 10 days.
> 2. Indep. transfers sit↔stand & on/off toilet within 10 days.

Anticipated Goals

1. Amb. c̄ walker 50% PWB Ⓡ LE for ~20 ft. ×2 within 5 days of Rx
2. Pt. will demonstrate transfers sit↔stand & on/off toilet c̄ min. assist +1 within 5 days of Rx
3. Pt. will demonstrate Ⓡ quadriceps strength of at least 2/5 within 5 days of Rx to assist. c̄ amb.
4. Pt. will indep. demonstrate exercises that he is to perform in his room within 2 Rx sessions

Intervention Plan: BID in dept.: amb. training c̄ a walker beginning c̄ 50% PWB Ⓡ LE & progressing wt. bearing & distance as tolerated. Transfer training sit↔stand, on/off toilet with emphasis on patient safety. Pt. will be given written & verbal instruction in exercise program to be performed in his room (attached). AAROM progressing to AROM exercises Ⓡ knee emphasizing quadriceps functioning. <u>Reaction to Rx:</u> AAROM exercises ×10 reps Ⓡ knee this date; Pt. was completely fatigued p̄ examination & initiation of exercise.

Writing the Intervention Plan

Here are some things to consider and include when writing the Intervention Plan.

Modalities:
    Which modality
    Where
    How long
    Intensity
    What position (one that is best, most comfortable)
Examples:
US: W/cm², time, where, position, reaction, coupling agent
Electrical stimulation: type of current, intensity, type of contraction, where, time, position
Ambulation:
    Distance
    Level of assistance
    Device(s)
    Time it takes to travel that distance
    Weight-bearing status
    Type of gait pattern/gait deviations noted
Exercise:
    Extremity or trunk
    Types
    Repetitions
    Position
    Equipment used
    Modifications

    Amount of resistance given (or weight used)
    Done in which planes
Home programs (usually attached to D/C notes as part of medical record):
Brief goal/rationale statement
    Illustrations
    Position
    Directions: keep language simple and in patient terms
    Repetitions and times/day to be performed
    Progression
    Equipment
    Precautions

A Word About Progress Notes and Revision

The Intervention Plan needs to be revised as the patient's condition is reexamined and reevaluated and new anticipated goals are set. When revision is necessary, the revision of the Intervention Plan is mentioned in a progress note, along with the changes noted during reexamination, reevaluation, and the resetting of anticipated goals.

A Word About Discharge Notes

Generally, the following should be briefly stated:

• the interventions the patient received
• if instruction in a home program was done, how well the patient performed the home program, the purpose of the home program, and the specific exercises included in the home program
• if any other type of instruction was performed and the result of this instruction
• if the patient was sold any type of equipment (e.g., weights, assistive device, lumbar roll), if the patient was instructed in how to use the equipment, and if the patient was independent in using the piece of equipment
• if a referral to a home health agency, another setting for therapy, or any other professional was made

If instruction of any kind is performed, the following information should be considered or recorded:

• *Who* was instructed (patient, patient's family member)
• The *type* of instruction (verbal, written, demonstration)
• The level of the patient or patient's family functioning (e.g., could independently demonstrate, could correctly describe the activity, could state the precautions needed for ADL)

The discharge note should also include the following information:

• The number of times the patient was seen in therapy
• If and when the patient was not seen/on hold and why

- Any instances of the patient skipping or canceling treatment sessions
- Where the patient is discharged (e.g., rehabilitation center, skilled nursing facility, home)
- The reason for discharge from therapy (goals achieved, transfer to another facility or type of therapy, patient requested discharge from therapy, patient illness, or death)
- Recommendations for follow-up treatment or care given to the patient

example

Intervention Plan: Pt. was seen BID for gait & transfer training to improve gait pattern, transfer sequence, & independence in ambulation & transfers. Pt. was also seen for (L) LE AROM exercises to hip, knee, & ankle joints in all planes of movement [initial date] through [discharge date]. Pt. refused Rx in P.M. of [date] & A.M. of [date] 2° severe nausea. D/C PT on this date p̄ 6 Rx sessions 2° D/C of Pt. from Hospital XYZ to home. Pt. & Pt.'s daughter were instructed in attached home exercise program for (L) LE AROM exercises & given a copy of same program & Pt. was indep. in same program. A folding walker was ordered for Pt. per Pt. request & walker was properly fitted to Pt. Pt. will be followed by ABC Home Health Agency for therapy to further progress Pt. toward expected outcomes for function in the home.

Summary and Objective

The Intervention Plan (P) part of the note is the final step in the planning process for patient care. In initial and progress notes, it outlines the interventions to be used with the patient. The interventions received on the date of the note and the reaction to these interventions are also listed. In discharge notes, it summarizes the interventions the patient received, the total number of intervention sessions, any patient education performed, handouts or equipment given or sold to the patient, and recommendations for future interventions or follow-up care.

The worksheets that follow give you the chance to identify Intervention Plan statements and to write the Intervention Plan portion of the note. For the purposes of this workbook, you are not expected to generate an appropriate Intervention Plan without guidance. After reviewing the previous information, completing the worksheets, and comparing your work to the answer sheets, you should be able to write the Intervention Plan part of the note if you are given the information to be included.

References

1. American Physical Therapy Association: Guide to Physical Therapist Practice, ed. 2, and CD-ROM. American Physical Therapy Association, Alexandria, VA, 2003.
2. American Physical Therapy Association: Defensible Documentation for Patient/Client Management. Accessed at http://www.apta.org/AM/Template.cfm?Section=Documentation4&Template=/MembersOnly.cfm&ContentID=37776 on March 9, 2007.

Writing the Intervention Plan

> **PART I.** Mark the statements that should be placed in the Intervention Plan by placing an *IP* on the blank line before each statement. Also, mark the Expected Outcomes by marking *EO* on the line before the statement, and indicate Anticipated Goals by marking an *AG* on the line before the statement.

1. _____ Will be seen 3×/wk. as an OP.

2. _____ ↑ strength (R) hip flexors, abductors & extensors to 3+/5 in 1 wk to assist Pt. c̄ progression toward indep. amb.

3. _____ Amb. training, working to ↑ wt. bearing (R) LE & ↓ gait deviations, progressing to uneven surfaces & obstacles.

4. _____ Pt. will be instructed in correct performance of AROM exercises (R) hip to ↑ (R) LE function during amb. & correct gait deviations.

5. _____ ↑ AROM (R) hip to 100° flexion in 1 wk. to progress Pt. toward indep. amb. & transfers.

6. _____ Strengthening exercises (R) hip musculature to ↑ indep. in amb.

7. _____ Pt. will be able to amb. on level surfaces c̄ a straight cane s̄ gait deviations in 1 wk.

8. _____ Pt. will be instructed in home exercise program to ↑ strength (R) hip musculature & ↑ AROM (R) hip for progression toward indep. amb.

9. _____ Pt. will be able to perform single leg stance on (R) LE for 10 seconds in 1 wk. to progress Pt. toward appropriate gait pattern.

10. _____ Pt. will be able to amb. s̄ assist. device FWB for 300+ ft. ×2 indep. around obstacles & including turns & ↑ & ↓ stairs in order to participate in his normal community activities p̄ 3 wks. of OP Rx.

> **PART II.** Write the following information into clear, concise statements regarding interventions (include verbs to make the phrases/sentences complete).

1. Hot pack—20 minutes—once per day—lumbar area to relax musculature prior to exercise

Answer: _____

_____

2. Continuous ultrasound—7 minutes—1.0 watts per centimeter squared—right upper trapezius muscle—three times per week

Answer: _____

_____

3. Twice per day at bedside—progress patient through exercise program of knee flexor and extensor strengthening exercises—attached—bilat. lower extremities

Answer: _____

_____

> **PART III.** Read each of the following Intervention Plans and state what is missing.

1. Pt will receive compression pump Rx.

Answer: _____

_____

2. Pt. will receive whirlpool BID.

Answer: _____

_____

Answers to "Writing the Intervention Plan: Worksheet 1" are provided in Appendix A.

Writing the Intervention Plan

> **PART I.** Mark the statements that should be placed in the Intervention Plan by placing *IP* on the blank line before each statement. Also, mark the Expected Outcomes by marking *EO* on the line before the statement, and indicate Anticipated Goals by marking an *AG* on the line before the statement.

1. _____ Training in floor↔stand transfers to assure safety in her home.

2. _____ Pt. will be able to amb. FWB c̄ walker indep. on level surfaces for 5 blocks including turns & obstacles, stairs, & uneven surfaces to reintegrate Pt. into the community p̄ 4 wks. of Rx.

3. _____ Pt. will be given a home exercise program for general LE strengthening.

4. _____ Pt. will be able to perform floor↔standing indep. to ensure Pt.'s safety at home & in the community within 4 wks. of Rx.

5. _____ Will be seen 3×/wk. in her home.

6. _____ Pt. will be able to perform sit↔stand transfers from a low chair indep. in 1 wk. to prepare Pt. for floor↔stand transfers.

7. _____ Pt. will be able to amb. c̄ walker 500 ft. indep. on level surfaces within her home, including turns, in 1 wk. to prepare Pt. for community amb.

8. _____ Pt. will ↑ LE strength to 4−/5 throughout bilat. within 1 wk. to improve amb. & floor↔stand transfers.

9. _____ Pt. will be able to amb. obstacles in her home c̄ walker indep. in 1 wk. to prepare Pt. for community amb.

10. _____ Amb. training FWB c̄ walker, beginning on level surfaces within the home & progressing to obstacles, stairs, & uneven surfaces.

11. _____ Pt. will be indep. in home exercise program for bilat. LE extensor strengthening within 1 wk. to assist. Pt. c̄ amb. & floor↔stand transfers.

PART II. Write the following information into the Intervention Plan part of the note.

---

1. Sue Smith will be seen three times per week as an outpatient. You will first give her a pulsed ultrasound to her right shoulder at 1.5 watts per cm² for seven minutes. She'll then get mobilization to her right shoulder. You'll end Rx c̄ an ice pack for 20 minutes. You also plan to teach her a home exercise program for AROM to the right shoulder to improve your patient's overall shoulder function. You plan to attach a copy of it to your note. You also will seek an OT referral for an ADL evaluation because she states she cannot do anything for herself at home.

INTERVENTION PLAN:

_____

_____

_____

_____

_____

_____

_____

_____

_____

_____

_____

2. Rodney Racecar will receive treatment twice per day at his bedside. He will be taught proper care of his residual limb and how to wrap his residual limb to prepare it for future ambulation with a prosthesis. He will receive resistive range of motion exercises to his legs beginning with 10 repetitions each and increasing the number of repetitions to 3 sets of 30 repetitions. The purpose of the resistive range of motion exercises is to prepare him for future ambulation. He will receive gait training with axillary crutches non-weight-bearing right leg and also transfer training sit to/from stand, on/off toilet, supine to/from sit to prepare the patient for independent functioning at home.

INTERVENTION PLAN:

_____

_____

_____

_____

_____

_____

_____

_____

_____

_____

_____

_____

Answers to "Writing the Intervention Plan: Worksheet 2" are provided in Appendix A.

Patient/Client Management Note: History, Systems Review, Tests and Measures, Evaluation, Diagnosis, Prognosis, Plan of Care
SOAP Note: Problem, S, O, A, & P

Begin by turning to the corresponding answer sheets at the end of these instructions so that you can write your Patient/Client Management Note and your SOAP Note directly on the answer sheets. A separate answer sheet is provided for each of the types of notes and is labeled accordingly.

The following are the notes to yourself that you jotted down while reading the chart, interviewing the patient, and performing the objective tests. (While taking notes for yourself, you did not consult Hospital XYZ's approved abbreviations list nor were you particularly careful in your notation style.) Take some time to read through the information below before writing your notes.

Make sure you begin your note by placing the date that you wrote the note on the first line, immediately prior to beginning the first section of the note.

FROM THE CHART

16 y.o. female

Pt. of Dr. Gungo

Fractured Right distal tibia and fractured right proximal humerus

ORIF Right proximal humerus on (date—yesterday)

Patient has a cast applied to the right leg and is in a sling for the fractured humerus

Patient is right handed.

Patient is currently taking [pain medication]—takes no other medications regularly

X-ray revealed good alignment of right lower extremity fracture in cast and good alignment of Right humerus after surgery.

From the Interview

The patient complains of pain in right ankle while in a dependent position (10 on a 0–10 pain scale) and severe pain (7 on a 0–10 pain scale) in right shoulder with elbow AAROM.

Lives c̄ both parents—1 story house—1 step at entrance with no handrail—has carpeting throughout.

Pt. was independent in ambulation and all of her activities of daily living prior to this accident

Never used a wheelchair before.

Pt. was in a car accident with one friend—friend was driving—friend is OK and in the community without injury at this time.

Is a high school student and wants to return to school as soon as possible after discharge.

School is on one level with no steps to enter the school. However, distances between classrooms are up to 1500 feet long. Has 7 class periods per day. All floor surfaces are linoleum.

School is very academically challenging and competitive and does not believe she can stay out of school until she is healed.

Parents attended therapy with patient; state their insurance will rent the patient a wheelchair.

Patient and parents report patient is an athlete—on swim team at school—generally good health—swims daily all year.

No previous hospitalizations or serious illnesses.

Does not smoke cigarettes or drink alcohol

Patient's parents both work so Pt. will be at home alone at discharge until she can go to school.

Pt. reports is having difficulty feeding herself and cannot dress herself. Has not seen OT.

Height: 5 ft. 6 inches, weight 125 pounds.

Family health history includes hypertension in both parents controlled by medication.

Systems Review

(Some of this information is drawn from the chart and from the previous interview—see these sections to complete the systems review.)

Cardiopulmonary not impaired

BP 110/70

HR 70

Resp. rate 12

Edema—none noted

Integumentary—impaired

Disruption of skin at incision site right upper arm

Continuity of skin color—bruising right upper extremity and right foot

Skin Pliability—normal left extremities; right extremities not tested this date

Musculoskeletal system—impaired

Gross symmetry—scannot stand; within normal limits in sitting

Gross ROM impaired right upper and lower extremities

Gross strength impaired right upper and lower extremities

Neuromuscular system

Gait impaired

Locomotion impaired

Balance not impaired in sitting and cannot stand

Motor function not impaired

Communication age-appropriate—not impaired

Oriented to person, place, and time/date—not impaired

Learning barriers: none

Pt. best learns: listening as she tries an activity

Education needs: healing process; adaptation of home to w/c; w/c management, w/c propulsion; ADLs; safety c̄ w/c; home exercise program for right upper extremity

Tests and Measures Performed

Bruising noted all of right upper extremity and on toes of right foot

Some bruising noted right posterior trunk

Left upper extremity—WNL AROM & strength

right shoulder not examined further due to recent fracture

right elbow AAROM is 30–70°

rigjt hand and wrist AROM very slow but WNL when patient is encouraged to complete full ROM—verbal cues are needed

right biceps & triceps strength is 2/5

Musculature controlling the right wrist and hand strength is 3/5

Left lower extremity—WNL AROM and strength

Right Lower Extremity—WNL at knee and hip—AROM

right Lower Extremity—strength 5/5 at knee and hip

right Lower Extremity—toes warm and normal color—able to wiggle toes

right Lower Extremity—short leg cast right ankle and foot so not further examined

Toilet transfers not tested today due to patient fatigue

Sit to and from stand with maximal +1 assist

Supine to and from sit with moderate assistance of one person

Wheelchair to and from bed with maximal +1 assist

Weight bear status is NWB right Lower Extremity

Weight bearing status is NWB right Upper Extremity

Cried when her right ankle was initially put in dependent position (pain level of 10)

right ankle pain level subsided after Pt. put right lower extremity in a dependent position multiple times

Unable to manage right wheelchair brakes, or leg rest

Propelled wheelchair ten feet using left leg and arm and was too exhausted to continue; required minimal assistance of 1 person and verbal cues to do so

> ■ **PART I.** Write a Patient/Client Management note using the pages provided to write the note.

Begin by writing about the examination. Don't forget to begin with the date you are writing the note. Write the History, Systems Review, and Tests and Measures parts of the note from the information initially listed.

Now write the Evaluation part of the note. You believe that rigorous AROM to the right elbow, wrist, and hand are needed to prevent them from losing strength and ROM. You also know that the patient's lack of mobility is due to her inability to use her right extremities due to her recent fractures. You also believe a referral to OT is essential to the Pt.'s rehab. process to assist her with eating, bathing, dressing, and managing items for return to school in a wheelchair.

Now write the Diagnosis part of the note. The patient's problems fall into Musculoskeletal Practice Pattern G: Impaired Joint Mobility, Muscle Performance, and ROM Associated With Fracture.

Now write the Prognosis part of the note. You believe that the patient has excellent rehabilitation potential. You believe that the patient will be able to return home and to school with 2 weeks of rehabilitation. You believe that the patient cannot stay at home alone after discharge until he or she becomes independent in wheelchair propulsion & transfers. You also believe the patient will need assistance in moving the longer distances in the school (more than 500 feet).

Now write the Expected Outcomes part of the note. You believe all of these expected outcomes will be achieved by discharge in two weeks.

1. Set the first expected outcome for transfers. You believe the patient will be independent in all of the transfers listed in the initial note (refer to the tests and measures part of the note). This will help the patient to be functional at home and at school. Write this information into expected outcome #1.

2. Set the second expected outcome for wheelchair management. You believe the patient will be independent in wheelchair management (brakes and footrests) to be functional at home and at school. Write this information into expected outcome #2.

3. You will set the third expected outcome for wheelchair propulsion. You judge that the patient will be independent in wheelchair propulsion for 500 feet twice in order to function at school. She will use her left UE and LE. Write this information into expected outcome #3.

4. You will set the fourth expected outcome for prevention of loss of function. You believe the patient will be able to prevent losing function in the right elbow, wrist, and fingers to maximize UE function when humerus is healed. Write this information into expected outcome #4.

Now set the anticipated goals.

1. Look at the first expected outcome. You think the patient will be able to transfer supine ↔ sit c̄ verbal cues by the end of 1 wk. Write this information into anticipated goal #1.

2. Continue to look at the first expected outcome. You think the patient will be able to transfer sit ↔ stand with minimal assistance of one person by the end of the first week of therapy. Write this information into anticipated goal #2.

3. Continue to look at the first expected outcome. You think the patient will be able to transfer w/c to and from the bed and on and off the toilet with moderate assistance of 1 person by the end of the first week. Write this information into anticipated goal #3.

4. Look at expected outcome #2. You believe the patient will be able to manage the brakes and footrests of the wheelchair using an extended brake lever on the right with verbal cues by the end of the first week of therapy. Write this information into anticipated goal #4.

5. Look at expected outcome #3. You believe the patient will be able to propel her wheelchair for approximately 100 feet with verbal cues by the end of the first week of therapy using her left arm and leg. Write this information into anticipated goal #5.

6. Look at expected outcome #4. You believe the patient be able to perform AROM to the right elbow, wrist, and fingers independently by the end of the first week to provide for right UE function after the patient's right humerus is healed. You believe the patient will be independent in performing a home program of AROM exercises to the right elbow, wrist, and fingers. Write this information into anticipated goal #6.

Now write the intervention plan for the patient.

• You plan to see the patient BID at bedside.

• You plan to instruct the patient in transfers (list all of the transfers listed in anticipated goals #1 through #3).

• You plan to instruct the patient in wheelchair management (see wheelchair details in anticipated goal #4). You plan to instruct the patient in wheelchair propulsion so she can be independent in her home and school settings.

• You plan to instruct the patient in a home exercise program for AROM to the right elbow, wrist, and fingers and give the patient a copy of the program. You plan to ask the patient to perform the program for you daily with supervision to ↑ AROM of her right elbow, wrist, and fingers and to perform the program by herself in her hospital room twice a day. You have attached a copy of the home exercise program to this note.

Sign the note (remember to use the appropriate initials behind your name).

Patient/Client Management Note

> **PART II.** Write a SOAP Note using the pages provided to write the note.

Begin by writing about the examination. Don't forget to begin with the date you are writing the note. Write the Problem, S, and O parts of the note.

Now write the A part of the note. Begin with the Evaluation. You believe that rigorous AROM to the right elbow, wrist, and hand are needed to prevent them from losing strength and ROM. You also know that the patient's lack of mobility is due to her inability to use her right extremities due to her recent fractures. You also believe a referral to OT is essential to the Pt.'s rehab. process to assist her with eating, bathing, dressing, and managing items for return to school in a wheelchair. Next write the Diagnosis Part of the note. The patient's problems fall into Musculoskeletal Practice Pattern G: Impaired Joint Mobility, Muscle Performance, and ROM Associated With Fracture. Continuing writing the A part of the note by writing the Prognosis. You believe that the patient has excellent rehabilitation potential. You believe that the patient will be able to return home and to school with 2 weeks of rehabilitation. You believe that the patient cannot stay at home alone after discharge until he or she becomes independent in wheelchair propulsion & transfers. You also believe the patient will need assistance in moving the longer distances in the school (more than 500 feet).

Next write the P, or Plan of Care, part of the note. Begin by writing the Expected Outcomes. You believe all of these expected outcomes will be achieved by discharge in two weeks.

1. Set the first expected outcome for transfers. You believe the patient will be independent in all of the transfers listed in the initial note (refer to the tests and measures part of the note). This will help the patient to be functional at home and at school. Write this information into expected outcome #1.

2. Set the second expected outcome for wheelchair management. You believe the patient will be independent in wheelchair management (brakes and footrests) to be functional at home and at school. Write this information into expected outcome #2.

3. You will set the third expected outcome for wheelchair propulsion. You judge that the patient will be independent in wheelchair propulsion for 500 feet twice in order to function at school. She will use her left UE and LE. Write this information into expected outcome #3.

4. You will set the fourth expected outcome for prevention of loss of function. You believe the patient will be able to prevent losing function in the right elbow, wrist, and fingers to maximize UE function when humerus is healed. Write this information into expected outcome #4.

Now continue the Plan of Care by setting the anticipated goals.

1. Look at the first expected outcome. You think the patient will be able to transfer supine ↔ sit c̄ verbal cues by the end of 1 wk. Write this information into anticipated goal #1.

2. Continue to look at the first expected outcome. You think the patient will be able to transfer sit ↔ stand with minimal assistance of one person by the end of the first week of therapy. Write this information into anticipated goal #2.

3. Continue to look at the first expected outcome. You think the patient will be able to transfer w/c to and from the bed and on and off the toilet with moderate assistance of 1 person by the end of the first week. Write this information into anticipated goal #3.

4. Look at expected outcome #2. You believe the patient will be able to manage the brakes and footrests of the wheelchair using an extended brake lever on the right with verbal cues by the end of the first week of therapy. Write this information into anticipated goal #4.

5. Look at expected outcome #3. You believe the patient will be able to propel her wheelchair for approximately 100 feet with verbal cues by the end of the first week of therapy using her left arm and leg. Write this information into anticipated goal #5.

6. Look at expected outcome #4. You believe the patient be able to perform AROM to the right elbow, wrist, and fingers independently by the end of the first week to provide for right UE function after the patient's right humerus is healed. You believe the patient will be independent in performing a home program of AROM exercises to the right elbow, wrist, and fingers. Write this information into anticipated goal #6.

Now complete the Plan of Care by writing the Intervention plan for the patient.

- You plan to see the patient BID at bedside.

- You plan to instruct the patient in transfers (list all of the transfers listed in anticipated goals #1 through #3).

- You plan to instruct the patient in wheelchair management (see wheelchair details in anticipated goal #4). You plan to instruct the patient in wheelchair propulsion so she can be independent in her home and school settings.

- You plan to instruct the patient in a home exercise program for AROM to the right elbow, wrist, and fingers and give the patient a copy of the program. You plan to ask the patient to perform the program for you daily with supervision to ↑ AROM of her right elbow, wrist, and fingers and to perform the program by herself in her hospital room twice a day. You have attached a copy of the home exercise program to this note.

Sign the note (remember to use the appropriate initials behind your name).

SOAP Note

_____

_____

_____

_____

_____

_____

_____

_____

_____

_____

_____

_____

_____

_____

_____

_____

_____

_____

_____

_____

_____

_____

_____

_____

_____

_____

_____

_____

_____

_____

_____

_____

_____

_____

_____

_____

_____

_____

Answers to "Final Review Worksheet" are provided in Appendix A.

V The Medical Record

*T*he evolution of medical records parallels advancements in medicine. The first incorporated hospital in America, Pennsylvania Hospital, was established in 1752. Benjamin Franklin served as the secretary for the hospital and recorded the patient's name, address, disorder, date of admission, and date of discharge on each patient. Massachusetts General Hospital in Boston has the distinction of having a complete medical record on each patient since 1821. In addition, Massachusetts General Hospital has used disease and operation data for research, statistics, and improving patient care.[1]

Today, technology affects all aspects of health care. The medical record is no exception. Hospitals and practitioners are moving from a paper-based record to an electronic health record. Whether paper-based or electronic, the medical record is the link connecting all of health care. The medical record is a valuable tool used by all entities involved in the provision of patient care including the practitioners, hospital, patient and family, and third-party payors. This section provides an overview of the purpose, maintenance, and content of the medical record, the legal aspects of the medical record, and the relationship between documentation in the medical record and reimbursement.

17 Overview of the Medical Record

Jody Smith, PhD, RHIA, FAHIMA

Purpose of a Medical Record

The medical record, paper-based or electronic format, should contain sufficient information to justify the patient's diagnosis, treatment, and services rendered. Documentation in the record should explain the patient's progress including the response to therapy, medication, or care rendered. Medical records play the following roles in supporting the health care industry[2]:

- serve as a communication tool that facilitates ongoing care and treatment of the patient
- justify reimbursement for hospitals and other health care practitioners
- serve as a legal document describing the health care services provided
- are a resource for research and education
- support clinical decision making
- provide information for the evaluation of the quality of care provided
- are a source of data for outcomes research

Maintaining a Medical Record

Medical records are maintained by all entities that provide health care to patients. Physicians, dentists, chiropractors, podiatrists, optometrists, nurses, physical and occupational therapists, hospitals, urgent care centers, rehabilitation centers, skilled nursing facilities, residential facilities, emergency care facilities, home health, behavioral health, and correctional facilities are required to maintain a patient's medical record. Documentation requirements and the type of record maintained vary according to the type of facility and provider. Information links all aspects of the health care delivery system, which underscores the need for all health care providers to document information to meet the needs of the patient and to comply with the laws and regulatory standards.[3]

Maintaining a medical record for patient encounters and documenting the care provided is mandatory. Over the decades, health care has become complex, resulting in the need to have documentation that is accurate, timely, and legible. Regulatory agencies such as the Joint Commission on Accreditation of Healthcare Organizations (JCAHO), the Commission on Accreditation of Rehabilitation Facilities (CARF), the Accreditation Association for Ambulatory Healthcare (AAAHC), the American Osteopathic Association (AOA), the National Committee on Quality Assurance (NCQA), and the American Accreditation Healthcare Commission (AAHC) are just a few of the accrediting agencies that have standards for medical records and documentation. Attaining accreditation signifies that the institution has made a commitment to having high standards for performance improvement and quality improvement.[4]

The federal government became more involved in health care in 1965 with the establishment of the Social Security Act of which Medicare was a component. Medicare is a health insurance program for persons over the age of 65, persons under the age of 65 with certain disabilities, and those individuals with end-stage renal disease requiring dialysis or a kidney transplant.[5] Standards for medical record content and documentation for federal patients are established by the Centers for Medicare and Medicaid Services (CMS), a division of the federal Department of Health and Human Services.

example

Standard

Content of the record: The medical record must contain information to justify admission and continued hospitalization, support the diagnosis, and describe the patient's progress and response to medications and services.[6]

Periodic reviews of medical records by the State survey agency occur to ensure compliance with Medicare Conditions of Participation. Failure to demonstrate compliance could negatively impact reimbursement to the provider and the health care facility.

States also have specific documentation requirements as part of their licensure process. These regulations usually are under the direction of the state Department of Health. Failure to comply with the regulations could result in closure of the health care facility.

Ensuring Quality Documentation

The therapist providing the care is responsible for making high-quality entries into the patient's health record. These entries must be timely, legible, and authenticated in accordance with the rules and regulations specified by the institutions in which the therapist works. Therapists will need to adhere to the documentation guidelines for their own profession. The following are documentation guidelines that all health care providers should follow.[2,3]

1. All entries in the medical record must be dated and signed with your name and professional designation to identify the author of the entry.
2. Entries in the medical record by graduates pending licensure or students in a physical therapy or physical therapist assistant program must be authenticated by a licensed physical therapist or physical therapist assistant when allowed by law.
3. Entries in the medical record cannot be erased or deleted. Corrections in a paper record are made by drawing one line through the error, leaving the incorrect material legible. The error should be initialed and dated so that it is obvious that it is a corrected mistake. If using an electronic medical record system, use the appropriate procedure for indicating that a change was made without deletion in the original medical record.
4. All entries in the paper medical record should always be made in black ink. Colors such as red, green, purple, and pink do not copy or scan well.
5. Blank spaces should not be left in the progress notes, treatment notes, or nursing notes. Record an "X" in the blank area to prevent the insertion of additional information that would be out of date sequence.
6. All blanks on consent forms should be completed.
7. Documentation should include the referral mechanism by which the physical therapist services are requested.

Locating Information in the Paper Medical Record

The medical record is a repository of data. Locating information in the paper record can be challenging. This section provides an overview of the contents of the patient's medical record to assist the therapist in pinpointing meaningful information.

Content of the Medical Record

The medical record contains two types of data—administrative and clinical. Regulatory agencies or professional organizations do not mandate a specific form. Form design is at the discretion of the health care organization or health care provider if working in private practice.

Administrative Section

Administrative data includes the patient's demographic information, such as name, address, date of birth, next of kin, payment source, billing or accounting number, and patient identification number, which is also called a medical record number.

Demographic information is collected at the time of registration and recorded on a face sheet or top sheet of the medical record. Facilities using a computer-based admission and discharge system will print out the demographic information on the face sheet or top sheet.

example
Demographic information must appear on each page of the patient's medical record. Therapists should verify that they are making entries in the correct medical record prior to making the entry.

Consent to release information, acknowledgment of patient rights, HIPAA acknowledgment, advance directives, consent to special procedures, property and valuable lists, and birth and death certificates are all considered administrative content.[2,3,7]

Clinical Section

Clinical content includes information related to the patient's condition, treatment, and progress. Clinical data makes up the majority of the medical record. Therapists must know each of the components of the clinical portion of the medical record to be able to find the information needed for patient care.

Medical History

The medical history and review of systems is the basis for formulating the provisional diagnosis and establishing a treatment plan. Contents of the history are somewhat subjective, since much of the information is provided by the patient or the patient's representative. Components of the medical history include the following[2,3]:

- Chief complaint (CC)—stated in the patient's own words explains why the patient is seeking treatment. Example: "My throat hurts."
- History of present illness (HPI)—describes the duration, location, and reason for the current condition.
- Past medical history (PMH)—documents any relevant childhood illnesses, previous surgeries, injuries, or illnesses that might have a bearing on the current condition. Allergies and drug sensitivities are also documented in the PMH.

- Social history (SH)—addresses habits, living conditions, occupation, marital status, psychosocial needs, alcohol consumption, and tobacco use.
- Family medical history (FMH)—documents conditions considered genetic or conditions of family members that might have relevance to the case such as diabetes, cardiovascular disease, or cancer.
- Review of systems (ROS)—asks questions that derive information that the patient might not have provided. All systems in the body will be inventoried. Information in this section is not to be confused with the results of the physical examination as performed by the medical practitioner.

Physical Examination

The physical examination provides objective data on the patient's condition. All body systems are included in the physical examination. There should be information in the record that addresses all the body systems with special emphasis on the areas that are pertinent to the Chief Complaint and the Review of Systems. A clinical impression and course of action based on the medical history and physical examination concludes the history and physical. The therapist will find the history and physical examination beneficial in obtaining sufficient information to assist in patient care.[2]

Interdisciplinary Patient Care Plan

The Patient Care Plan lays the foundation for the care provided to the patient. Each discipline associated with the patient contributes to the Patient Care Plan, which includes an assessment of the patient, statement of desired goals for the patient, strategies on attaining the goals and a periodic assessment of progress made toward achieving the goals. The Patient Care Plan is reviewed at scheduled intervals and revised as needed.[2]

Physician or Practitioner Orders

The Joint Commission defines a licensed independent practitioner (LIP) as, "any individual permitted by law and by the organization to provide care, treatment, and services without direction or supervision."[7] As a therapist, it is important to determine your level of authority in writing orders by checking the facility's policies and procedures, as well as the bylaws, rules, and regulations of the medical staff.

Orders communicate the type of treatment and diagnostic procedure(s) the practitioner wants for the patient to carry out the care plan. Orders can be verbal or written. Verbal orders must be authenticated in accordance with state and federal regulations; bylaws, rules, and regulations of the medical staff; and regulatory agencies. Use of standing orders is discouraged because not all of the actions on the standing order may be medically necessary for the patient.[2,3]

Progress Notes, Patient/Client Management Notes

Notes are interval statements that relate to observations about the patient's progress and response to treatment from the perspective of the professional. How often notes are written depends on the patient's condition. Therapists need to document every visit or encounter. Documentation should include what was done including frequency, intensity, and duration as appropriate, equipment provided, changes in the patient/client treatment plan, reaction to the treatment, and communication with the patient/client/family or other health care providers.[2,3]

> example
>
> In addition to dating and authenticating your progress note, some facilities require that you provide a start and stop time documenting when you were with the patient. This will be important when billing for services rendered to the patient. Remember: Write your professional credentials after your signature.

Consultation

A consultation report contains an opinion about a patient's condition by a practitioner other than the attending physician. It is important for the consultant to document their opinion based on a review of the patient record, examination of the patient, and conference with the attending physician. Consultants address their specialty area only.[2,3]

Discharge Summary, Clinical Resume

For patients who have a medical record from a prior admission available, the discharge summary or clinical resumé summarizes the patient's course in the hospital or other care setting. This is a great place to find significant findings from examinations, laboratory tests, procedures, and therapies along with how the patient responded. The patient's condition on discharge, physical activity, diet, medications and follow-up care are included in the discharge summary.[2]

Pertinent information can be found elsewhere in the medical record including in the operative report, pathology report, nursing notes, medication record, laboratory reports, radiology and imaging reports, radiation therapy, and notes from therapists such as speech, occupational therapy, physical therapy, respiratory therapy, and dietetics.

> example
>
> Remember, the medical record is a communication tool. Although abbreviations, acronyms, and symbols save time when documenting, they can be misinterpreted by others, placing the patient at risk. If your facility has an approved abbreviation list, be sure to use only those abbreviations exactly as they appear in the approved list. The Joint Commission has a list of abbreviations that are not to be used in the medical record. The list can be accessed at http://www.jointcommission.org/ NR/rdonlyres/2329F8F5-6EC5-4E21-B932-54B2B7D53F00/0/06_dnu_list.pdf

Electronic Health Record (EHR)

Health care facilities are beginning to transition from a paper record to one that is computer-based, or electronic. The EHR is a repository for all the patient data collected from components of the electronic systems, such as computerized physician order entry, laboratory, pharmacy, radiology, imaging, admissions, and transcription. The EHR provides the caregivers, the patient, and others with access to patient-specific information or information on a group of patients for research purposes.[2]

Summary and Objective

Information contained in the medical record links all of health care. The value of the medical record to the care providers and institution is only as good as the documentation in the record. Therapists must take the initiative to follow the documentation guidelines specified in the rules and regulations where they work. Remember: Write legibly and make timely entries in the medical record. The EMR is being implemented throughout the health care industry. Good documentation habits should be carried over to the EMR as well.

References

1. Huffman, E, and Cofer, J (eds): Health Information Management. Physicians' Record Company, Berwyn, 1994.
2. Abdelhak, M, et al: Health Information: Management of a Strategic Resource. Saunders, St. Louis, 2007.
3. LaTour, K, and Eichenwald-Maki, S: Health Information Management: Concepts, Principles, and Practice, ed. 2. AHIMA, Chicago, 2006.
4. Carol, R: Accreditation: The First layer of the quality floor. Journal of AHIMA 73(1):22–26, 2001.
5. Medicare Program General Information. Accessed at http://www.cms.hhs.gov/MedciareGenInfo/ on June 5, 2007.
6. Condition of Participation: Medical Record Services. Accessed at http://www.access.gpo.gov/nara/cfr/waisidx_04/42cfr482_04.html on June 5, 2007.
7. Joint Commission on Accreditation of Healthcare Organizations: 2005 Comprehensive Accreditation Manual for Hospitals. JCAHO, Oak Brook Terrace, 2005.

18 Legal Aspects of the Medical Record

Jody Smith, PhD, RHIA, FAHIMA

*T*he medical record is a legal document that is admissible as evidence in a court of law. As a health care professional, you have the responsibility to keep health information accurate, secure, and confidential.

Keeping the Record Secure

Securing the medical record involves minimizing the chance of getting a record lost, altered, damaged, or destroyed.

> **example**
>
> Ways to secure a paper record include:
> - controlling access to the file room
> - keeping records under lock and key
> - not leaving records lying around
> - developing and adhering to policies and procedures pertaining to physical threats such as fire, water damage, and natural disasters[1]

In 1996, Congress passed the **Health Insurance Portability and Accountability Act (HIPAA).** The Administrative Simplification provisions of HIPAA required the Department of Health and Human Services (DHHS) to establish national standards for the security of electronic health care information. This final rule specifies a series of administrative, technical, and physical security procedures for covered entities to use to assure the confidentiality of electronic protected health information.

> **example**
>
> Ways to protect electronic health care information include[2]:
> - limiting access to information through the use of passwords, key cards, or biometric identification
> - restricting copying function
> - including security mechanisms in contracts with outsourced vendors
> - establishing policies addressing the use of laptops and personal digital assistants
> - using time out monitors
> - developing a disaster recovery plan

Confidentiality

Health care professionals are bound by law and ethical standards to maintain the confidentiality of private health information. Confidentiality means protecting patient-specific health information from disclosure.[2]

The APTA Guide for Professional Conduct section 2.3 discusses confidential information. Physical therapists directly treating patients and physical therapists performing a peer review function may not release the patient's information to anyone who is not directly involved in that patient's care without obtaining prior consent of the patient. The exception to this would be disclosure of information to authorities for purposes of protecting the welfare of an individual or community or as mandated by local, state, or federal law.[3]

> **example**
>
> **2.3 Confidential Information**
> A. Information relating to the physical therapist/patient relationship is confidential and may not be communicated to a third party not involved in that patient's care without the prior consent of the patient, subject to applicable law.
> B. Information derived from peer review shall be held confidential by the reviewer unless the physical therapist who was reviewed consents to the release of the information.
> C. A physical therapist may disclose information to appropriate authorities when it is necessary to protect the welfare of an individual or the community or when required by law. Such disclosure shall be in accordance with applicable law.

Health information is confidential and privileged and therefore cannot be disclosed without specific authorization from the patient or as authorized by law or by a court. An authorization to release information should be in writing (Fig. 18-1), but can be via a computer if allowed by state law. The following elements constitute a valid authorization to release information[2]:

1. Name and identifying information of the person providing the authorization

PRETTY GARDEN
MEDICAL CENTER

AUTHORIZATION FOR RELEASE OF HEALTH INFORMATION

UNIT NUMBER

PT. NAME

BIRTHDATE

LOCATION   DATE

I authorize _____
Name of person or facility which has the information

to release health information to:

_____
Name of person or facility to receive health information

_____
Specify name/title of person to receive health information (if known)

_____
Street Address, City, State, Zip Code

_____
Fax Number (if information is to be faxed)

The purpose of this release is for (check one or more):

☐ Continuity of care or discharge planning

☐ Billing and payment of bill

☐ At the request of the patient/ patient representative

☐ Other (state reason) _____

_____

Please specify the health information you authorize to be released:

Type(s) of health information: _____

Date(s) of treatment: _____

The following information will not be released unless you specifically authorize it by marking the relevant box(es) below:

☐ Information pertaining to drug and alcohol abuse, diagnosis or treatment (42 C.F.R. §§2.34 and 2.35).

☐ Information pertaining to mental health diagnosis or treatment (Welfare and Institutions Code §§5328, et seq).

☐ Release of HIV/AIDS test results (Health and Safety Code §120980(g)).

☐ Release of genetic testing information (Health and Safety Code §124980(j)).

EXPIRATION OF AUTHORIZATION

Unless otherwise revoked, this authorization expires_____(insert applicable date or event). If no date is indicated, the authorization will expire 12 months after the date of my signing this form.

_____
Print Name

_____
Date   Time

_____
Signature (Patient, Parent, Guardian)

_____
Relationship to Patient (Parent, Guardian, Conservator, Patient Representative)

_____
Witness (only if patient unable to sign) or Interpreter

AUTHORIZATION FOR RELEASE OF HEALTH INFORMATION

Fig. 18-1. Sample Release of Information form

2. Name of the institution authorized to release the information
3. Name of the institution or person to whom the information is to be released
4. Specific description of what is to be released
5. Date the authorization expires
6. Statement of the individual's right to revoke the authorization and the exceptions to the right to revoke the authorization
7. Statement informing the patient that the information being released may be redisclosed and may lose its protected status
8. Signature of the individual and the date signed
9. If authorization is signed by someone other than the patient, the relationship of the individual to the patient

Health information management professionals have expertise in the security, confidentiality, and privacy of medical records and patient information and can be a valuable resource for legal matters pertaining to the medical record.

S u m m a r y   a n d   O b j e c t i v e

The medical record is a legal document that can be subpoenaed and used as evidence in a court of law. All health care professions have the responsibility to protect the privacy and confidentiality of the patient's information.

Each state has specific rules addressing how to keep health information accurate, secure, and confidential. Congress established national standards for securing electronic health care information. These standards are referred to as the Health Insurance Portability and Accountability Act (HIPAA).

Physical therapists can refer to the APTA Guide for Professional Conduct for details on what patient information can or cannot be released to requesting individuals. Another resource often overlooked is the health information management professional who has expertise in the security, confidentiality, and privacy of medical records and patient information.

R e f e r e n c e s

1. Abdelhak, M, et al: Health information: Management of a Strategic Resource. Saunders, St. Louis, 2007.
2. McWay, D: Legal Aspects of Health Information Management, ed. 2. Thomson Delmar, New York, 2003.
3. APTA Guide for Professional Conduct. Accessed at http://www.apta.org/AM/Template.cfm?Section=Core_Documents1&Template=/CM/HTMLDisplay.cfm&ContentID=24781 on June 6, 2007.

19 | Reimbursement

Jeanne Donnelly, PhD, RHIA

Reimbursement involves the health care provider, the patient, and the third-party payor. The third-party payor is an individual or insurance organization that is responsible for paying the patient's bill for the health care encounter. The medical record is used to justify reimbursement to the health care facility, health care provider, or both. Documentation in the medical record is reviewed, coded, and entered into a billing system. Once a patient has been seen by a practitioner, the process of reimbursement begins. There are several different payment methodologies depending on the setting and the type of insurance that the patient has. This section will outline the basic steps in the reimbursement process.

Coding the Information

Code numbers are a communication link between the health care provider and/or health care facility and the third-party payor. Every diagnosis and procedure that the patient receives requires a numerical code number. There are numerous coding systems in use today, but the United States primarily uses ICD-9-CM (International Classification of Diseases, 9th Revision, Clinical Modification) and CPT-4 (Current Procedural Technology).

Codes should be assigned by a health information management (HIM) professional who has received extensive training in using the coding system. The HIM professional will assign code numbers based on the documentation in the medical record. Reimbursement is driven by the code numbers assigned. Without good documentation allowing the appropriate code numbers to be assigned, providers will not receive appropriate payment.

example

Inpatient

| Discharge Diagnosis: | Herniated disc, L4 | ICD-9-CM Code: 722.10 |
| Procedure: | Lumbar laminectomy | ICD-9-CM Code: 80.51 |

example

Outpatient

Diagnosis:	Herniated disc, L4	ICD-9-CM Code: 722.10
Procedure:	PT Evaluation	CPT Code: 97001
	Whirlpool Treatment	CPT Code: 97022

A **chargemaster** or **charge description master (CDM)** lists all the items that can be billed to a patient. Many of these items are tied to the ICD-9-CM and CPT-4 code. Among other elements, the file contains a code number, a description of the code, and the charge for the procedure or item. This information is tied to the billing system to ensure that the appropriate charges are filed for the procedures. When the code is entered, the corresponding charge appears on the patient's bill.

example

Charge Description Master

CPT CODE	DESCRIPTION	CHARGE
99203	Office visit, new patient	$250.00
97001	PT Evaluation	$238.00
97116	Gait Training with evaluation	$ 59.00

Billing for Service

The most common claim forms used by health care providers are the CMS-1500 for outpatient treatment and the UB-04 for inpatient treatment. Medicare requires the use of these forms, and most commercial insurance companies accept and use them. Copies of these forms can be found at https://www.bcbswy.com/providers/pdf/cms1500sample.pdf and http://www.ub04/net.

The billing forms capture demographic information about the patient and his or her insurer. The provider must enter information regarding the date of treatment, name of the physician or provider, the diagnosis, treatment, procedures, code numbers, and charges. The hospital bill will include charges for room and board, pharmacy, central supply, and other items that incur a charge during the hospital stay. When complete, the information is transmitted to Medicare, Medicaid, or another insurance provider. The payor then processes the claim and will issue payment to the provider based on prevailing rate or the rate that was negotiated between the payor and the provider. These forms cannot be processed without the appropriate ICD-9-CM or CPT-4 code numbers.

Getting Reimbursed

In 2005, 46% of the health care dollar came from government-sponsored programs. Medicare accounted for 17%, Medicaid represented 16%, and other public spending such as the Veterans Administration, worker's compensation, and Department of Defense provided 13% of the total dollar amount spent on health care.[1] The total amount of money spent on health care in 2005 was almost 2 *trillion* dollars.[2] The federal government has developed a payment methodology in an effort to control some of the health care costs.

Medicare

Medicare is a federally funded health insurance program developed for individuals over the age of 65, individuals under the age of 65 with certain disabilities, and those individuals suffering from end-stage renal disease.[3] Part A of Medicare covers the hospital charges for inpatient care, hospice care, and some home health care. Part B of Medicare covers physician services and outpatient care, including physical and occupational therapy. Part D of Medicare is the prescription drug coverage for Medicare beneficiaries.[4]

Medicaid

Medicaid provides medical benefits for low-income individuals. This program is jointly funded by the federal government and individual states. The requirements for Medicaid vary from state to state, but are tied to federal guidelines related to poverty limits. Medicaid funds may cover inpatient hospital stays, outpatient care, screenings for children, and some physical and occupational therapy.[5] The exact coverage is determined by the individual states. Both the Medicare and Medicaid programs are run through the Centers for Medicare and Medicaid Services (CMS).

Payment Methodologies

Inpatient Prospective Payment System (IPPS)

The federal government reimburses hospitals using Diagnostic Related Groups (DRG). Hospitals are reimbursed a set amount per DRG for care rendered to a patient. DRGs are defined by the type and amount of resources that are consumed by the patient during his or her stay. Information from the patient's chart is coded using the ICD-9-CM coding system. That information is entered into a computer program that groups or assigns a patient to a DRG based on the diagnosis and procedure. The reimbursement amount is determined by a combination of each individual hospital's rate, which is based on the case mix index, and the CMS weight of each DRG. Other factors that influence the reimbursement amount include the wage index for the local hospital, whether it is an urban or rural hospital, and whether it is a teaching hospital.

For example, a patient who has congestive heart failure and a cardiac catheterization would be grouped into *DRG 124: circulatory disorders except AMI, with cardiac catheterization and complex diagnosis.* The CMS weight

for DRG 124 is 1.4099. If Memorial Hospital's rate is $2063, the reimbursement rate for this patient would be $2909 *(1.4099 × 2063)*. Memorial Hospital would receive $2909 in reimbursement for each patient who was grouped into DRG 124. This payment does not include any reimbursement for physician services. It is only the hospital portion of the patient's bill. If a patient incurred more than $2909 in costs, the hospital would take a financial loss from the patient's stay. If the patient incurred less than $2909, the hospital would make a profit.

In 2008, Medicare will roll out a new version of the IPPS. Reimbursement will be based on DRGs that have been adjusted for severity. This new version will be called MS-DRGs (Medicare Severity Diagnostic Related Groups). MS-DRGs are based on the presence or absence of major and minor complications or co-morbid conditions. For example, in the MS-DRG system, heart failure will be categorized into three MS-DRGs:

MS-DRG 291: heart failure & shock with major complication/co-morbidity
MS-DRG 292: heart failure & shock with minor complication/co-morbidity
MS-DRG 293: heart failure & shock without major or minor complication/co-morbidity

The reimbursement rate for these MS-DRGs will be adjusted based on the severity of the patient's condition.

Outpatient Prospective Payment System (OPPS)

The federal government reimburses hospitals for ambulatory care using Ambulatory Payment Classifications (APC).[6] As with Diagnostic Related Groups, APCs are similar clinically and in terms of the number of resources they consume. Patient information is coded using the CPT-4 and HCPCS coding system. The reimbursement rate is determined by the CMS weight for each APC multiplied by a national conversion factor. Unlike the inpatient prospective payment system, in which a patient is assigned to only one DRG, a patient may have more than one APC assigned per visit. The number of APCs depends on the type of service and treatments the patient received during his or her visit.[7,8]

For example, a patient who came to the ambulatory center of Memorial Hospital for an arthroscopy may have two APCs—*APC 0041: Level I arthroscopy* and *APC 0607: Hospital Clinic Visit, Level IV.* The 2008 weight for APC 0041 is 28.7803, and the weight for APC 0607 is 1.6604. The national conversion factor for 2008 is $63.694. The hospital would be reimbursed $1883 (28.7803 × 63.694) for the arthroscopy and $105 (1.6604 × 63.694) for the visit for a total of $1938. These amounts are adjusted by the wage index.

Resource Based Relative Value Scale (RBRVS)

Physicians are reimbursed on a different payment schedule. Each CPT code is evaluated on three different components or Relative Value Units (RVU): the work involved, the practice expense, and the malpractice cost associated with the procedure. Each of these factors is multiplied by a geographic factor to account for the differing regional costs. This number is then multiplied by a conversion factor to determine the amount of reimbursement the physician practice will receive. The conversion factor for 2008 is $38.087.[9]

Based on the above formula, the amount of reimbursement for a PT evaluation in St. Louis, Missouri, is $74.04. The same evaluation in New York City would be $87.22.

Commercial Insurance

All three payment systems discussed above are for federally funded patients. Some commercial insurers abide by these methodologies, but in most situations, the commercial insurer bases payment on one of the methods below.

Negotiated Rate. Insurance companies will evaluate the usual, customary, and reasonable charges (UCR) for the area. When that is established, a rate is negotiated between the provider and the insurance company. Since historical and comparative information is used, it is crucial that the patient's medical record contain accurate documentation so that the appropriate rates and charges can be established.

Per Case. Rather than negotiate a rate for each specific patient, commercial insurers use a rate based on case. Examples of cases might be major and minor surgery,

cardiac surgery, pregnancies, and newborns. The types of patients included in these categories are identified through ICD-9-CM codes. Since these codes are based on the documentation in the chart, it is important that the caregiver document all treatments given to the patient.

Per Diem. Insurers may also negotiate a per diem, or per day, rate. In that case, hospitals would be reimbursed at a set cost per day. Different units might command different per diem rates. For example, the per diem rate for an intensive care unit would be higher than that for a regular floor.

Per Visit. Physicians, or ambulatory facilities, could negotiate a per visit rate. Physicians may be reimbursed one amount for an established patient and a higher reimbursement amount for a new patient. A per visit rate may also be used to reimburse for rehabilitative services. The insurance provider might evaluate the number of visits required for a patient after hip surgery and state that they will pay a certain amount for 10 visits.

Regardless of the type of reimbursement methodology used, the key is documentation. Patient charts are reviewed for the number and types of services performed, the length of stay, the diagnoses, Plans of Care, and other documentation that provides a total picture of what constitutes quality care. The better the documentation, the better a hospital, physician, physical therapist, or other practitioner can justify charges.

example

Physician Reimbursement

CPT Code	Description	Work RVU	Practice RVU	Malpractice RVU
97001	PT Evaluation	1.20	.73	.05
97024	Diathermy	.06	.07	.01
97116	Gait Training	.40	.25	.01

Geographic Index

St. Louis	1.00	.956	.926
New York City	1.052	1.283	1.756

Source: 2007 National Physician Fee Schedule Relative Value File, Centers for Medicare and Medicaid Services, www.cms.gov

S u m m a r y   a n d   O b j e c t i v e

Documentation and coding drive the reimbursement system for a hospital, a clinic, or a physician's office. Without proper documentation, HIM professionals cannot code the patient's chart accurately. If the information is not coded properly, the provider will not get the proper amount of reimbursement.

ICD-9-CM and CPT-4 are classification systems used to code patient information. In general, Medicare and Medicaid use three different payment methodologies for health care: MS-DRGs are used to reimburse hospitals for inpatient care, APCs are used to reimburse hospitals for outpatient care, and RBRVS is used to reimburse physicians. Commercial insurers may opt to use that methodology, but most reimburse using a negotiated payment schedule based on the usual, customary, and reasonable charges for the area, a per case basis, a per diem rate, or a per visit basis.

References

1. http://www.reimbursementcodes.com/hcpcs_codes_d.html
2. http://www.cms.hhs.gov/NationalHealthExpendData/downloads/PieChartSourcesExpenditures2005.pdf
3. http://www.cms.hhs.gov/NationalHealthExpendData/downloads/proj2006.pdf
4. http://www.cms.hhs.gov/MedicareGenInfo/
5. ibid
6. http://www.cms.hhs.gov/MedicareGenInfo/
7. http://www.cms.hhs.gov/HospitalOutpatientPPS/
8. http://www.cms.hhs.gov/hospitaloutpatientpps/downloads/cms-1501-cn.pdf
9. http://www.cms.hhs.gov/PhysicianFeeSched/

VI | Applications of Documentation Skills

Congratulations! You have mastered the skill of documenting patient care. Now that you have mastered the skills involved in documentation, a brief discussion of applications of documentation skills is needed. Applications of note writing and alternative formats to the Patient/Client Management Note and SOAP Note formats are presented (Chapter 20). Alternatives to writing notes, such as documentation forms and computerized documentation, are discussed (Chapter 21).

20 | Applications and Variations in Note Writing

This workbook has covered the reasons for writing notes and a brief history of the origins of the two note formats. It has offered a test of your working knowledge of medical terminology and a good review of abbreviations.

As you begin to practice in clinical settings, you will find that nobody writes patient care notes exactly as you were taught to write notes. Each facility that uses the Patient/Client Management or SOAP Note format has its own variations of the format. Within any facility using a set note format, each therapist has his or her own variations of the format used by the facility.

Applying the Patient/Client Management Note to Other Note Formats

Many facilities do not use the Patient/Client Management Note format at all. Some facilities use a single narrative style format. Others use an outline format of some kind. Still others (especially private practice settings) may send letters to the patient's physician describing the patient's condition, goals, plans, and so forth. School settings and chronic care settings may set yearly goals as part of a student's or patient's individualized education plan (IEP). Whatever format you may encounter, your knowledge of writing Patient/Client Management Notes should be helpful.

Narrative notes frequently include the same information used in the Patient/Client Management Notes, but the information may be in a different order.

Outline note formats, or *fill-in-the-blank forms,* also include the information that the note formats in this book contain. The information may be organized in a different order, and periods or sentences may not be used, but the information is still present. As long as you know how to organize the information and put the information into the categories used in the Patient/Client Management Note format, you only need to learn where to put the information in an unfamiliar format or form.

Letters written to a physician's office on a regular basis are also usually organized in a particular style to save time. Certain categories are placed in a certain order, according to the standards set forth by the physical therapy practice involved. If you know the categories of the note formats taught in this workbook, you will be able to rearrange them to fit into a letter format. However, caution should be taken in using letters as a therapist's only documentation of care. Letters are not written after each therapy session, and letters are not considered true documenation of patient care.

IEPs also have a standardized format that takes the information involved in the note formats taught in this workbook and renames and rearranges the categories. Goals that are set yearly become the Expected Outcomes. Whether or not they are officially written, Anticipated Goals to be achieved by different times during the year are set to meet the Expected Outcomes. The goal format taught in this workbook is very adequate for use in most educational settings.

Finally, not every facility that writes Patient/Client Management or SOAP Notes includes every part of the note formats covered in this workbook. Many facilities include the Expected Outcomes and Anticipated Goals in the *A* part of the note. Others combine the *A* and *P* portions of the note and list each Expected Outcome, the corresponding Anticipated Goal(s), and Intervention Plans together before moving on to the next problem. There are as many variations in note writing formats as there are facilities that offer therapy.

Uses in Clinical Decision Making

One of the reasons that the note writing formats that you learned in this workbook are so adaptable to other styles of note writing is that they represent more than simple documentation formats. They represent a method of clinical decision making. Although you were not expected to independently write the Evaluation, Diagnosis and Prognosis, set Expected Outcomes or Anticipated Goals, or generate Intervention Plans in this workbook, you were given many examples of how Patient/Client Management Notes and SOAP Notes can be used to plan a patient's care. As long as you use the note formats for yourself in approaching and solving patient problems, you can learn to write the information in any form that you might like.

A Word to the PTA or COTA

Many of the examples in this workbook included writing an entire initial patient care note. According to the standards of the professions, PTAs and COTAs do not write initial notes. However, the skills that you used to write the initial notes in this workbook can be used in writing progress notes in your daily practice. Many facilities ask the assistant to write the progress note and to document the goals and interventions set by the therapist and assistant together for their patients. One of the ways in which you can be most helpful to the therapists with whom you work is to assist them with the documentation included in patient care. Therefore, it is important that your skills in this area continue to be used and improve long after you no longer need this workbook.

Documenting All Types of Patient Care

Most of the cases used in this workbook were very simple. Some of your instructors may disagree with the method of documenting the details of the cases listed within this workbook. (For example, there are quite a few acceptable methods of documenting AROM.) As you approach learning while in school and throughout your career, be aware of the methods available to document what you learn, no matter what the subject matter. Ask your instructors how they document the information that they are teaching you. Ask for definitions of terminology such as *minimal, moderate,* and *maximal* as you begin to practice in various clinical facilities. It is important that you keep abreast of research into therapy tests and measures and use the most reliable, evidence-based scales.

As professions, physical and occupational therapy have done much to standardize terminology used in documentation, but they still have much do to in this area. Many facilities do not have written definitions for commonly used terms, such as physical assistance given.

Your experience in writing notes and documenting what you do as a therapist has barely begun with the completion of this workbook. You have learned to write Patient/Client Management Notes and SOAP Notes, to organize the information into categories within each section of the note, to be clear and concise in what you say, and to use abbreviations and medical terminology well. The application of the information is now up to you.

As with any skill, the continued use and practice of note writing will perfect your skills. You will adapt all that you have learned about writing notes to the style of each facility in which you practice. Eventually, even if you practice in a facility with a particular note-writing style, you will develop a style that is unique to you. You can develop expertise in documentation and help move the profession toward more standardized methods of evaluation and documentation.

In the immediate future, you may wish to remove the appendices from this workbook and keep them available as quick references on documentation. They summarize some of the information included in this workbook. They can assist you in applying what you have learned about writing notes as you continue the process of developing yourself as a member of the health care team.

21 Alternatives: Documentation Forms, Medicare Forms, and Computerized Documentation

As trends in health care change, documentation changes. Health care professionals are constantly looking for more efficient and effective ways to ease the task of documentation without losing their ability to act as professionals. Therefore, systems of documentation that can be performed at the point of care have been developed at some facilities and are currently being developed by other health care facilities and outside companies. As these processes were beginning, Medicare developed Forms 700 and 701 for purposes of obtaining consistent data that can help Medicare reviewers determine the appropriateness of the care given to patients.

Well-written Patient/Client Management Notes, SOAP Notes, documentation forms, Medicare forms, and computerized documentation share one characteristic: They provide structure to documentation. Structured documentation guarantees the collection of a consistent data set that can give us information about the outcomes and effectiveness of the interventions that we give our patients. Without this type of information, we will not be able to meet the challenges of managing both the cost and quality of health care delivery. Computerized documentation, including APTA CONNECT,[1] and tools, such as OPTIMAL,[2] can assist us in gathering the consistent data needed for our profession to progress.

Medicare Forms

Medicare developed Forms 700 and 701 in an attempt to gather consistent data needed to make decisions about whether the patient's condition and interventions qualify for Medicare coverage. Before these forms were developed, reviewers for Medicare were receiving poor-quality patient notes, some without goals, some without a good description of the patient's functional deficits. Medicare forms ask for (1) demographic information (the patient's name, age, and Social Security or Medicare number), (2) basic medical data (date of surgery or onset of condition, diagnosis), and (3) data that should already be contained in a well-written Patient/Client Management Note or SOAP Note. The data they request include functional status prior to therapy interventions and current functional status, long-term goals (expected outcomes), short-term goals (short-term goals, or anticipated goals, are listed as monthly goals), treatment (intervention) plan, and justification for treatment. It is easy to include the information required by these forms because the categories are similar to those of any good Patient/Client Management Note or SOAP Note. Medicare forms were never intended to replace documentation into the medical record; their intended use was to gather consistent data on Medicare patients.

Documentation Forms and Computerized Documentation Programs

In some facilities, forms are used for documentation or documentation is done on the computer. Facilities usually have unique documentation forms or some type of computerized documentation format. The purpose of this section is to review some advantages and disadvantages of each of these formats for documentation and to include items for consideration when developing forms or considering the purchase of a computerized documentation system.

Documentation Forms

Documentation forms are used in many clinics for many reasons. Some of the reasons include the following:

- decreasing the amount of writing by the therapist/assistant
- increasing the efficiency of the therapist/assistant in documenting patient care
- increasing the consistency of documentation (and thus fulfilling certain quality assurance or legal/risk management requirements) by building certain components into a note, such as whether the patient is given a home program, and his or her level of independence in performing the home program
- making the data gathered for outcomes studies more consistent
- making functional information easier to read by all parties who use the information

Forms are usually individualized to fit the needs of the individual health care institution and its patient population. When designing a form, it is helpful to watch how clinicians practice. Forms should include the items that the therapist commonly examines. Other additions to the forms can be obtained by asking staff members to use the forms and give feedback to those designing the forms.

When beginning to use a new form, it is important for the therapist/assistant to give himself or herself time to adapt to the use of the form. Becoming familiar with the form before seeing a patient makes the therapist much more efficient in the use of the form.

The most efficient use of a form is to complete the form, or at least begin its completion, while seeing the patient. If you can write your examination findings directly on the form, you will save time. *Caution:* Do not let the use of forms limit your practice! If an item is missing from a form, find a place to write it (if it is relevant to the patient's function). Forms should have a place for the therapist to write observations and analyses that may be an exception to the norm of patients in a diagnostic group. Also, forms should be revised on a regular basis to meet the needs of good clinical practice.

Types of Documentation Forms

Several types of documentation forms are in use in various facilities. These include the following:

- Flow sheets
- Initial examination/discharge note forms
- Progress/discharge note forms
- One-visit-only documentation forms
- Supplemental forms to be attached to initial, progress, or discharge forms (often have specialized tests or scales that are needed only for certain types of patients)

Development of Documentation Forms

When developing a form, take the following into consideration:

- Do not reinvent the wheel unless you really must. Revising a form from another facility (used with permission, of course) is much easier than starting with nothing.
- When you have developed a draft version of the form, ask yourself and those who must use and read the form if the form does what it is supposed to do for all parties involved (health care providers, those concerned with reimbursement, and so on).
- Communicate with all parties involved when you develop forms. If the form is to be useful, everyone must know how to use the form (both writing on the form and reading the form).
- Examination items frequently used by the staff should be included following the patient/client management process.[3,4]
- If a standard scale, test, or definition of measurement is used by all staff to measure or document a certain

characteristic of the patient or a certain facet of patient care, a checklist may be faster in documenting the test or measurement.

- Checklists can save the therapist time because they speed up documentation.
- If you use any sort of checklists in your note forms, try to make the checklists consistent or similar from one form to another. This saves confusion and unnecessary staff reorientation time.
- Frequently leave space for very brief comments or descriptions.
- Unless the form is created with a very specific patient population in mind, allow for a general examination of the patient.
- If there are no standardized methods of documenting the information derived from your examination of the patient, allow room for writing.
- Forms influence practice, so be sure to include items that you believe are essential to practice.
- If the staff has been writing Patient/Client Management Notes or SOAP Notes, transition for the staff will be easier if you follow a similar format. Because these formats support clinical decision-making, documentation using this type of format will assist the staff in clinical decision-making.
- Function should still be stated first in the tests and measures portion of the note form, just as you should do so when writing notes.

Computerized Documentation

Computerized documentation continually changes and develops as technology improves. Some facilities have a well-developed program that is tailored to the needs of that facility. Within the past few years, many improvements will be seen in the area of computerized documentation, including software that precisely follows the Patient/Client Management Note format in its output of data.[1] This section will serve as a review of some of the features that have been developed or are in stages of development by various companies and health care systems throughout the country.

The advantage of computerized documentation over the use of forms is that the limitations of paper become unimportant because the computer is not limited to any particular size in which to place the information gathered. Computers can also have all of the possible tests and measurement available, so the therapist is not limited by the tests and measurements available on a given form.

Some features that will make computers even easier to use in the future are the following:

- *Data can be entered by making choices and simply touching a stylus to the screen or clicking a mouse. This* makes data entry more consistent and does not require advanced keyboard competence.

- *Data can be printed in a variety of formats.* Information can be printed in the formats required or requested by any insurance carrier and in the format of a Patient/Client Management Note for the medical record. It could also allow the therapist to choose certain functional or relevant data to send to the patient's physician or other referral source, as needed.
- *The medical record can be retrieved and notes written at the patient's bedside.* Some health care facilities have computers located in every patient's room or between every two rooms. With notebook and pocket-sized computer technology available, the therapist is able to have a notebook with him or her that contains or can access the medical record and rehabilitation information for all the patients the therapist treats.
- *All documentation can be completed at bedside.* Even outpatient and home health care therapists are able to have the computer with them and complete all documentation while they work with the patient. Notebook and pocket-sized computers with removable keyboards are already available.
- *Handwriting recognition is a feature that has been developed and will continue to be developed in the next few years.* This enables the therapist to enter extra notes and information as needed (much as therapists now do when they use forms and need to remark about the unusual quality of a movement), although many therapists prefer using a keyboard to writing.
- *Voice recognition is a feature that continues to be developed.*[5] This could completely change our methods of data entry, although some caution must be taken in the use of voice-activated methodology while at the patient's bedside.
- *Charging will be able to be done by the therapist immediately upon completing the patient's care and while she or he completes other computerized documentation (and the computer may remind the therapist to charge the patient).* Computerized charging systems exist in many

clinics today. Moving the charging to the patient's bedside, along with all other documentation functions, will greatly increase therapist efficiency and relieve the repetition in documentation that some therapists experience today.

When looking at computerized documentation systems, items that deserve consideration are listed in the following text:

- It is important to consider the needs of therapists at their individual practice sites. A system should be flexible enough to fulfill the needs of the therapist at the individual practice site; otherwise, the system is not worthwhile.
- Computerized documentation systems vary in their mobility, weight, flexibility, ease of use, speed of data entry, and speed of the hardware. All of these factors must be considered when purchasing or developing a computerized system. Compatibility with the patient/client management model[3,4] and the potential for collecting data for outcomes studies must also be considered.[1,2]
- Training time must be taken into consideration when you discuss the cost of a computerized documentation system. A system that requires extensive training must also save much time to be cost-effective.
- Technology is worthwhile only if it makes the therapist's task of documentation easier and allows her to do something she could not do without the technology. For example, the time spent documenting should be decreased, and spelling errors or obvious errors in recording of data should be pointed out to the therapist automatically for the purpose of immediate correction.
- The willingness, availability, and cost of programmers to customize the system to the individual facility's needs should be investigated before making a commitment to a computerized documentation system. If the computerized documentation system used is commercial, the amount of support and times that support is available must be considered.

Summary and Objective

Many facilities have developed documentation forms to help therapists document faster and more efficiently. Forms must be developed by a facility's therapists to meet their practice needs.

Computerized documentation will be the primary mode of documentation in the future and is already used in many facilities today. Just as documentation forms must be customized to the practice at an individual practice site, computerized programs must be customized to meet the needs of therapists at an individual site.

Forms and computerized documentation do not exclude the type of thinking that is used in note writing. As mentioned previously, the Patient/Client Management Note and SOAP Note formats help therapists structure their thinking about patient problems and the attainment of the patient's goals for function. As forms and computer programs are further developed, aspects of clinical decision-making will continue to be used to help the therapist meet patient needs while he or she documents.

References

1. Waldrop S: APTA Connect: Software for improved patient documentation and outcomes measurement. PT Magazine, October 2006.
2. Guccione, A, et al: Development and Testing of a Self-Report Instrument to Measure Actions: Outpatient Physical Therapy Improvement in Movement Assessment Log (OPTIMAL). Physical therapy, June 2005.
3. American Physical Therapy Association: Guide to Physical Therapist Practice, ed. 2, and CD-ROM. American Physical Therapy Association, Alexandria, VA, 2003.
4. American Physical Therapy Association: Defensible Documentation for Patient/Client Management. Accessed at http://www.apta.org/AM/Template.cfm?Section=Documentation4&Template=/MembersOnly.cfm&ContentID=37776 on March 9, 2007.
5. Voice Recognition Goes Home. Health Management Technology; January 2003.

22 The Future: Documentation Using the International Classification of Functioning, Disability and Health (ICF) System

Theresa Bernsen, PT, MA

*E*xperienced rehabilitation specialists know that a person's medical diagnosis does not always provide a predictable picture of how a person functions in daily life. Imagining a person with a medical diagnosis of "stroke" or "osteoarthritis" can conjure images of different levels of function that cannot be explained by the severity of the diagnosis alone. Other factors such as the accessibility of the person's environment, the person's financial status, and the strength of his or her social support system can create significant differences in functional outcomes. The World Health Organization's (WHO) International Classification of Functioning, Disability and Health (ICF) seeks to avoid the pitfalls of disability models that describe a person's health status based on one feature, such as medical status or societal attitudes. The ICF framework uses a "biopsychosocial" model of health that acknowledges the interaction of biological, social, and personal factors to provide a more nuanced description of an individual's health experience.[1,2]

ICF Informs Medical Documentation

Description or classification of a person's health status using ICF is based on the multi-factoral framework shown in Figure 22-1.[1]

All of the factors or classifications surround the factor of "Activity," which is defined as the execution of a task or action by an individual. A person's ability to perform activities is presumably affected by all the factors that surround it. "Participation" appears as a factor distinct from activity and is defined as involvement in a life situation. However, field usage and the evolving ICF literature illustrate some tendency to treat the two factors of activity and participation as one factor: Activity and Participation. There is some concern about the practical usefulness and need to differentiate the two factors.[2–6] The ICF text provides hundreds of examples of activity and participation, with several chapters providing descriptions of tasks with significant motor components.

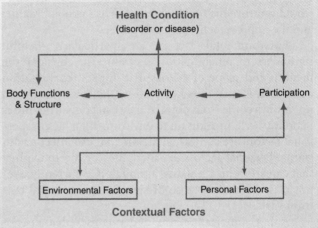

Fig. 22-1. ICF Framework

Descriptions of motor tasks vary widely, from maintaining a body position such as sitting or kneeling to more high-level tasks such as running, swimming, preparing complex meals, and the acquisition of goods.[2]

The factor of health conditions represents diseases or medical disorders. The factors of body functions and body structures account for the physiologic and anatomical status of the body. Body functions refer to physiologic descriptions and are inclusive of the all body systems. Again, a wide variety of descriptors are available, such as psychomotor control, visuospatial perception, the perception of pain, vestibular function, and various aspects of cardiovascular and respiratory function. Muscle and joint functions, such as mobility of particular bones, the power and endurance of particular muscles, the status of reflexes, and resting muscle tension, are a few of the many body functions that will sound familiar to rehabilitation specialists. Body structures refer to the status of anatomical features of the body in every organ system. Discrete structures of the brain, spinal cord, heart, respiratory system, integumentary system, bones, joints, and ligaments are described.[2]

207

Contextual factors include both environmental factors and personal factors. Environmental factors describe the person's physical environment, such as the availability of food, drugs, products, technology for personal use (e.g., chairs, tools, appliances); assistive products for personal use (e.g., prosthetic and orthotic devices, remote controls, wheelchairs); financial assets; and building design. Environmental factors also include the societal expectations and attitudes in which the person is immersed, which is an area that health professionals do not always formally recognize in documentation.[2] An example of an environmental factor relating to societal expectations that would influence the health status of a person would be the parents of a child who uses a wheelchair who do not expect people with disabilities to participate in sports. The child's ultimate health status could be impeded because his caregivers do not allow him to participate in exercise that would improve his health status such as aerobic training and the improvement of muscle power.

Environmental factors are particularly helpful reminders to rehabilitation specialists to consider the breadth and scope of factors that impact rehabilitation outcomes. Constraints imposed by the environment do not always come from objects; they can come from other people as well. In addition to environmental factors, personal factors are contextual factors that can affect health status. Personal factors are attributes of the individual that can affect health status, although ICF currently does not classify these because of significant social and cultural variances.[2]

A few important terms and premises that do not appear in the ICF framework itself need to be understood within its context. "Impairments" are problems with body functions or structures. Problems with activities are "activity limitations," and problems with participation are "participation restrictions." Things that promote a positive health status in environmental factors are "facilitators" and things that impede health status are "barriers." In ICF, "disability" takes on a broad meaning to include impairments in body function or structure, as well as activity limitations and/or participation restrictions. Problems with body functions and body structures and/or activities and participation are based on deviations from generally accepted population standards of people without health conditions. Remember that in ICF, a disability does not necessarily provide a predictable decline in health status. Things such as environmental factors, personal factors, and the severity of the disability or health disorder will influence the ultimate outcome of a person's health status.[2]

create a particular person's health status. It is the first health model to have significant input into its formation by representatives of people with disabilities as well as people related to the provision of health care.[2,7] Accordingly, ICF emphasizes that information gathered in a person's health record about environmental factors is just as relevant for understanding a person's health status as a medical diagnosis. This reason alone would justify its use.

In addition to the advantages for describing health status, ICF is becoming an integral part of medical documentation and research. The National Committee on Vital and Health Statistics (NCVHS) has recommended ICF's terminology, classification systems, and conceptual framework as a "common language" for electronic information exchange across federal agencies as part of the Consolidated Health Informatics (CHI) Initiative.[8,9] This recommendation has received the support of the Department of Health and Human Services (DHHS), which means that ICF language will be incorporated into the U.S. National Library of Medicine's Unified Medical Language System.[10,11] The DHHS is associated with significant federal agencies as diverse as the Social Security Administration (SSA), the Veteran's Administration (VA), the Centers for Disease Control and Prevention (CDC), the National Center for Health Statistics (NCHS), the National Institutes of Health (NIH), the National Center for Medical Rehabilitation Research (NCMRR), and the Centers for Medicare and Medicaid Services (CMS).

While ICF is becoming an integral part of communication within federal health agencies, it is also becoming embedded in exchanges of health information throughout the world. An important example is WHO's plans to link ICF to its classification system for medical diagnostics, the International Classification of Disease (ICD). ICD is the international standard diagnostic classification used for epidemiological and other health management purposes. Plans for creating the latest iteration of ICD, the ICD-11, include aligning ICD-11 with the ICF classification system. ICF's "health conditions" factor offers a natural connection to ICD-11. Such a connection encourages components of health status found in ICF to be included in the description of ICD diagnostic categories, and will facilitate information processing about a broader range of health status issues related to the diagnostic category. Explicit relationships between ICF and ICD will encourage the exchange of health-related information, particularly within electronic applications for public health purposes and other forms of health-related research.[12,13]

Why is ICF Important for Medical Documentation?

ICF obviously gives clinicians a more realistic, integrative model for thinking about all the factors that converge to

ICF Does Not Replace Diagnostic Labels Specific to a Profession

Because many of the categories under body functions, body structures, and activities and participation contain terms that are familiar to rehabilitation specialists, it is easy to confuse ICF's classification system with a diagnostic labeling system that is particular to a profession such as physical therapy. Remember that the purpose of ICF is to provide a universally understood description of health status. The language of ICF is intentionally "profession neutral," so that all professions may use the ICF system to describe health status. For example: the category of walking found under activities and participation can be used to help describe the effects of interventions from a wide variety of professions. Orthopedists can use the walking classification to describe the success of particular kinds of surgical interventions. Neurologists can use the same classification to describe the success of pharmacological intervention. Physical therapists can use the classification to describe the effects of rehabilitation or changes in a person's environment. This profession-neutral approach encourages multi-professional and inter-professional approaches to the resolution of disability.

Because ICF is profession neutral, there may be useful descriptors of health status that an evaluator would like to provide, but are not included in the current list of categories available in ICF. This is why all categories in the three classifications of body functions, body structures, activities and participation, and environmental factors include options for categorization called "other, specified." The other, specified categories allow an evaluator to provide further description about health status by assigning a label to a new category. The other, specified categories may evolve into a description used only by certain groups of evaluators for particular purposes, or have such universal utility that it could become its own category in the next edition of ICF. For example, the current category of walking does not include a category that describes velocity; a feature of walking that can have a significant impact on disability.[2] Interested parties could agree on standards for categorizing walking velocity and use the d4508 other, specified category. If the successful utility of the other, specified category is shared with other users of ICF, the options for useful descriptors of health status will grow. This potential for organic growth is why particular groups who use ICF but do not find a category that represents a potentially useful descriptor, should make a concerted effort to use the other, specified category rather than ignore the deficit.

ICF Framework and Prognosis: A Model That Illustrates Paths to Disability, Prevention, and Wellness

Recall that the ICF framework (see Figure 22-1) contains multiple categories that describe all of the factors that join together to affect a person's health status. Because each factor is joined to the others with arrows, it is easy to see how a health condition such as rheumatoid arthritis can cause impairments in body functions and body structures such as impairments in the structure of the hand and mobility of several joints. These impairments will lead to limitations in preparing simple meals, a category in activities and participation. Without successful intervention at the level of the environment, such as assistive products and technology, or resolution of impairments in body structure and function, the person will experience disability. In this manner, the ICF framework describes a frequent prognosis—that those with health disorders often experience some level of disability via impairments in body structure or function and/or through activity limitation/participation restriction. However, two visual features of the ICF framework remind us of more complex relationships among ICF categories: ICF's nonlinear structure and its use of bidirectional arrows.

The nonlinear structure of the ICF framework reminds us that a problem in one category does not inevitably lead to problems in another category. Interconnected arrows allow the evaluator to reach one category while bypassing or modifying another. A person may experience the health condition of occlusion of cerebral arteries, which in turn causes impairments in the power of muscles of one side of the body. While most people who experience this health condition have a poor prognosis for the activity of walking long distances, this is not true of everyone. Impairments in muscle power may be so minimal that they do not cause a limitation in the activity of walking long distances. Environmental factors such as assistive products or technology for personal indoor and outdoor mobility can also change the person's prognosis for activity to a more positive one. The nonlinear structure is a visual reminder that not all health conditions result in disability and that, in some cases, a particular prognosis is not inevitable.

Secondly, ICF's use of bidirectional arrows joining each component serves as a visual reminder that we can also describe how impairments in body functions and body structures can lead to limitations in activities and participation, and in turn exacerbate a health condition. For example, a person with impairments in the power of muscles in all limbs may be unable to perform activities under the category of changing and maintaining body position. In turn, this person may suffer impairments in skin structure due to lack of mobility, resulting in loss of the protective function of the skin and exacerbation of the health conditions of decubitus ulcers and infection. However, if the person lives in an environment with supportive relationships with immediate family who are willing to assist the person in turning and positioning methods to prevent impairments in skin structure, the ICF framework can illustrate a positive prognosis resulting from the interventions that promote the person's wellness.

The visual features of the ICF framework are a tremendous boon to professions who want to illustrate how their interventions can not only improve disability, but prevent further exacerbation of disability and worsening of health conditions through services aimed at prevention and wellness. The ICF framework reminds us that a person's prognosis could be a description of increasing disability, or in the best of scenarios, the decreasing of disability and severity of health conditions and the promotion of well-being.

ICF Coding: Classification and Description of a Person's Health Status

For ease of communication, ICF describes the state of a person's health status in its various classifications or domains by using a coding system made up of groups of letters and numbers. The four domains classified by ICF are represented by letters:

- Body Functions (b)
- Body Structures (s)
- Activities and Participation (d)
- Environmental Factors (e)

In turn, each domain has numerous descriptors called categories, which are represented as a number following the domain's letter representation. For example: coding a person's range of motion of her scapula would be coded as "b7200," where "b" represents the domain of body functions and "7200" the particular category of mobility of the scapula. The present status of a category is always described through the use of qualifiers that are represented by numbers that appear after a decimal point in the code. In the case of the person with limited range of motion in her scapula, we can use a generic scale for the qualifier to describe the extent of the impairment. A generic scale for severity may be as simple as the numbers 0-4, with 0 representing no impairment, 1 representing the mildest impairment (5-24% loss of range of motion), and 4 representing a complete loss of range of motion (96-100% loss of range of motion).   If the person in our example has completely lost all range of motion of her scapula, the information would be conveyed by the ICF code of "b7200.4." The number of qualifiers that appear after the decimal point, as well as the scales chosen, can be tailored to fit the purposes of the coding. While members of the ICF community are creating standard sets of qualifiers, new groups of qualifiers can be created to meet future demands for health-related information.[2]

When coding, all domains and categories must have qualifiers that appear after the decimal point. It is the qualifiers that describe the actual status of the category. Not to include qualifiers in a code would be the same as stating that a person can run, but not describing how fast or how far; stating that a person has broken his or her tibia, but not indicating how severely or what kind of fracture; or stating that a person lives in a dwelling, but not indicating whether it is a shelter made of sticks or a penthouse apartment. In this sense, coding has a clinical relationship with the examination and evaluation of a person.

To help learn coding practices, the ICF community is assembling clinical companion manuals to supplement the ICF text. These manuals, both for the standard ICF text and the pediatric version, are titled: *Procedural Manual and Guide for Standardized Application of the ICF: A Manual for Health Professionals.*[14] Ease of use is also promoted by breaking ICF categories into user-friendly subsets of codes designed for particular professions or for describing people with particular health conditions. "Core sets" are subsets of codes created to describe people with particular health conditions. There are core sets in development for a wide variety of health conditions, including stroke, rheumatoid arthritis, low back pain, and breast cancer to name but a few.[15] Other "code sets" can be created to provide the codes most germane to a profession, such as a set of codes that a physical therapist is most likely to use in daily practice.

ICF and Expected Outcomes

The *Guide to Physical Therapist Practice* recommends that expected outcomes be written in functional terms.[16] ICF categories listed under the classifications of activity and participation contain resources upon which the therapist can draw for ideas about functional outcomes related to motor performance. These chapters include activities that frequently appear as expected outcomes in rehabilitation, such as transfers, maintaining sitting and standing, ambulation, wheelchair use, carrying objects, preparing meals, and performing various kinds of self-care and household tasks. There are other activities that are less commonly thought of as outcomes, such as pushing or pulling objects, climbing, using transportation such as bicycles, driving a car, the acquisition of goods and services, and caring for household objects (e.g., cars, plants, animals). There are even categories for people who need to perform activities to be caretakers for others in the household. Other major areas include activities for educational and employment settings, participation in religion and spirituality, and recreational and leisure activities.[2] The activities and participation classification provides a rich resource for therapists to expand their ideas about what constitutes a functional outcome. Conversely, therapists who establish an outcome for an activity that is not included in the current list of ICF categories should write the outcome using one of the other, specified categories. In this manner, outcomes that are specific to a group of interested parties can gather data on the outcome, and new ideas with potential for high utility can be introduced in later versions of the ICF.

Outcomes have another relationship with ICF through the coding system used for activities and participation, and in particular, through the use of qualifiers. Figure 22-2 shows a model of a code for the category of walking short distances in the domain of activity and participation.

The first four qualifiers for activity and participation are used to describe a person's current abilities under different conditions. Qualifiers that use the term "performance" are descriptions of how well the person walks in daily life situations in their typical environments, such as their home or neighborhood. Qualifiers that use the term "capacity" are meant to convey the person's highest probable level of ability in a standardized environment such as a clinical setting. Describing the person's abilities in standardized environments is an attempt to remove the varying environmental factors that are impeding the person's best possible performance.

In this case, the first qualifier "performance" is a rating of how well the person performs walking in his or her usual environment. The second qualifier "capacity without assistance" is a rating of how well the person performs the same task of walking in a standardized environment, such as a clinic, but without direct assistance from a person or device. The third qualifier "capacity with assistance" rates how well the person performs walking in the same standardized environment with the assistance of a person or devices. The fourth qualifier "performance without assistance" rates the person's ability to walk in his or her usual environment, but without the assistance of people or devices.[2]

If we consider a person who is having difficulty walking short distances, the evaluator can illustrate differences in performance of this activity under different conditions through the use of performance and capacity qualifiers. Below is an abbreviated scale of the qualifiers used for the activity of walking short distances (less than a kilometer).

d4500 Walking Short Distances

0   No limitation (0% to 4%, none)
1   Mild limitation (5% to 24% slight)
2   Moderate limitation (25% to 49%, medium)
3   Severe limitation (50% to 95%, high)
4   Complete limitation (95% to 100%, total)[2]

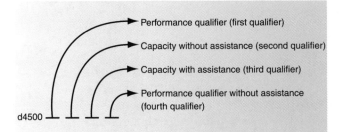

Fig. 22-2. Model of an activity and participation code identifying qualifiers

For example, if a person lives alone in a house with carpeting on the floor and no assistive device, she might score a "4" on the first "performance" qualifier because she cannot walk at all in her home environment. If she could walk in your clinic on an uncarpeted surface that would not impede her walking, but requires physical assistance of another to walk to any distance without a device, she would score a "4" on the second "capacity without assistance" qualifier. However, if given a quad cane and asked to walk on uncarpeted surfaces in the clinic, she can walk 10 feet independently. This would give her a score of a "3" for the "capacity with assistance qualifier." To illustrate the vital importance of assistive devices for this woman to improve her ability to walk, she would receive a "4" on the qualifier "performance without assistance" because she would again be unable to walk at all in her home environment without the quad cane. All of this information about her activity status for walking in all four of these scenarios would be summarized by the following ICF code: d4500.4434.

Differences in ratings among these four qualifiers can help clinicians demonstrate that by adding the assistance of a person or equipment or by changing environmental barriers, the patient's ability to walk short distances can improve. Information that shows improvement in the patient's status by coding the qualifiers in the activity and participation categories reinforces the positive achievement of outcomes in the patient's usual environment if appropriate assistance, equipment, and environmental changes are provided. Demonstrating such changes in health status through ICF coding is a way to reinforce the need for intervention to improve outcomes and to enhance patient advocacy.

ICF and Anticipated Goals

The *Guide to Physical Therapists Practice* describes anticipated goals as including function and/or impairments.[16] Goals that are functional and serve as steps along the way to achieving a functional outcome can use the same resources in the activity and participation chapters of the ICF that were mentioned for outcomes. Goals that are impairment based can be referenced to the chapters associated with body functions and body structures. Body functions categories listed under the chapters dealing with sensory function and pain, cardiovascular and respiratory systems, neuromusculoskeletal and movement-related functions, and functions of skin and related structures are categories with common and obvious uses for rehabilitation specialists, although most categories in body functions can be associated directly or indirectly with various aspects of motor performance.

While the status of body structures will obviously affect the prognosis for successful goals in rehabilitation, categories that describe impairments of body structures will probably be less frequently associated with clinically measurable goals in rehabilitation. Some body structures that may be helpful for goals are the categories for particular muscles and other soft tissues, particular joints (depending on how standards for description are developed), and parts of the integumentary system such as skin. Therapists who establish a goal for a body functions or body structures that is not included in the current list of ICF categories should write the goal using one of the other, specified categories. In this manner, goals that are specific to a group of interested parties have a way to be included in data analysis, and new ideas with potential for high utility can be introduced in later versions of the ICF.

Similar to outcomes, goals that address the resolution of impairments of body functions or body structures can be reinforced by documentation provided by ICF coding. The example below shows the use of a body function code "b7302" describing "power of muscles on one side of the body" and a scale for the first qualifier that denotes the severity of the impairment:

b7302.1 = mild impairment of power of muscles of one side of the body (5% to 24%)

b7302.2 = moderate impairment of power of muscles of one side of the body (25% to 49%)

b7302.3 = severe impairment of power of muscles of one side of the body (50% to 95%)

b7302.4 = complete impairment of power of muscles of one side of the body (96% to 100%)[2]

An absence of impairment below the criteria for "mild impairment" would be denoted as a "0" in the first qualifier.[2]

Documenting this ICF code for muscle power on different dates can show a progression in the person's ability to produce muscle power through changes in the first qualifier, and further support the documentation of goal achievement. For example, a person whose muscle power on the left side of the body is improving over time with rehabilitation might be coded b7302.3 (severe impairment) at the time of the initial evaluation; 3 weeks later, the person might receive a code of b7302.1 (mild impairment). Coding for impairments in body structures may also be used to provide reinforcing documentation for the achievement of goals.

Summary and Objective

ICF provides rehabilitation specialists the opportunity to describe multiple factors that influence the health status of the people they serve in an integrated fashion. ICF provides a context and a language for data concerning the services rehabilitation specialists provide for incorporation into various local, state, federal, and international health provision systems. ICF provides methods of describing the benefits of rehabilitation services for inclusion in the public health domain and various forms of research. Rehabilitation specialists need to become familiar with ICF, and participate in its ongoing development, if they are to participate effectively in all of these aspects of health and wellness services.

References

1. Towards a Common Language for Functioning, Disability, and Health . Accessed at: http://www.who.int/classifications/icf/site/beginners/bg.pdf on January 12, 2008.
2. ICF: International Classification of Functioning, Disability and Health. World Health Organization, Geneva, 2001.
3. Blending Activity and Participation Sub-Domains in ICF. Accessed at: http://www.cdc.gov/nchs/data/icd9/icfnov07newsltr.pdf on January 12, 2008.
4. Jette, AM, Tao, W, and Haley, SM: Blending activity and participation sub-domains in ICF. Disability and Rehabilitation 29(22): 1742–1750, 2007.
5. Schuntermann, M: The implementation of the International Classification of Functioning, Disability and Health in Germany: Experiences and problems. International Journal of Rehabilitation Research 28(2):93–102, 2005.
6. Perenboom, R, and Chorus AM: Measuring participation according to the International Classification of Functioning, Disability and Health (ICF). Disability & Rehabilitation 25(11-12):577–587, 2003.
7. DPI Position Paper on Definition of Disability. Accessed at: http://v1.dpi.org/lang-en/resources/details.php?page=74 on January 15, 2008.
8. National Committee on Vital and Health Statistics, Consolidated Health Informatics: Standards Adoption Recommendations. Accessed at: http://www.ncvhs.hhs.gov/061128lt.pdf on January 15, 2008.
9. Consolidated Health Informatics. Accessed at: http://www.hhs.gov/healthit/chi.html on January 20, 2008.
10. North American Collaborating Center ICF Newsletter, November, 2007. Accessed at: http://www.cdc.gov/nchs/data/icd9/icfnov07newsltr.pdf on January 15, 2008.
11. Letter from Secretary of Health and Human Services dated July 31, 2007. Accessed at: http://www.ncvhs.hhs.gov/070731lt.pdf on January 15, 2008.
12. Production of ICD-11: The Overall Revision Process. Accessed at http://www.who.int/classifications/icd/ICDRevision.pdf on January 13, 2008.
13. International Classification of Diseases. Accessed at http://www.who.int/classifications/icd/en/index.html on January 13, 2008.
14. NACC Clearinghouse ICF Messages November 2003. Accessed at: http://www.cdc.gov/NCHS/data/icd9/icfnov03.pdf January 22, 2008.
15. First Version of ICF Core Sets for Chronic Conditions. Accessed at: http://www.icf-research-branch.org/research/cc_icf_core_sets.htm on January 22, 2008.
16. American Physical Therapy Association: Guide to Physical Therapist Practice, ed. 2, and CD-ROM. American Physical Therapy Association, Alexandria, VA, 2003.

ICF Practice Case

You are a physical therapist in an outpatient facility. You receive a physician's order to "evaluate and treat" a person named Sophia who reports *shoulder pain*. Her physician has decided that she has *an impingement syndrome of her rotator cuff*. After several medical examinations, the physician reports that she also *has a partial tear of the supraspinatus tendon*. Sophia reports *a "stabbing" shoulder pain* that becomes severe when she attempts to raise her arm past shoulder height. She is having increasing difficulty taking care of herself and her home because she cannot perform such tasks as *combing her hair* or *washing her windows*. She is *unable to reach objects on the shelves of her kitchen cabinets*, although *she can reach the shelves in your clinic* because they are lower than her cabinets at home.

Sophia has been *unable to work for the last few months at her job as a factory worker* and is on leave from work. Her employer resents that she is receiving "workman's comp." payments. *Her employer refuses to let her return to work on a part-time basis because he feels she is exaggerating the amount of shoulder pain she experiences.* Sophia feels she could return to work full time if her employer would agree *to reconfigure her work station by lowering it. Her work station is currently too high for her to reach without shoulder pain.*

You notice that when you attempt to raise her arm overhead, Sophia displays *deficits in passive mobility of glenohumeral flexion.* Upon manual muscle testing, you note *the loss of power in all the abductors and lateral rotators of the glenohumeral joint.* Using several intervention techniques, Sophia recovers fully. In fact, her shoulder feels so much better, she decides to leave her job as a factory worker and resume a previously abandoned career as a tennis pro. Sophia goes on to win fame and fortune at Wimbledon, thanks to your skills.

Answer the following questions concerning the above case using the ICF terminology listed below:

activities and participation
b
activity limitation/participation restriction
body function
body structure
capacity qualifier
health conditions
d
disability
e
environmental barrier
environmental facilitator
environmental factor
impairments
performance qualifier
s

1a. If you use the ICF coding system to code *combing her hair* and *washing her windows,* in what domain would you find this code? _____

1b. What letter would represent this domain in the code? ___

2. She has been *unable to work for the last few months at her job as a factory worker.* The italicized phrase represents a(n) _____.

3a. If you use the ICF coding system to code *the loss of power in her abductors and lateral rotators of the glenohumeral joint,* in what domain would you find the code? _____

3b. What letter would represent this domain in the code? ____

4a. The *partial tear of the supraspinatus tendon* would be coded under what domain? _____

4b. What letter would represent this domain in the code? _____

5. Her *deficits in passive mobility of glenohumeral flexion, loss of power in all the abductor and lateral rotator muscles of the glenohumeral joint, "stabbing" shoulder pain* and *a partial tear of the supraspinatus tendon,* are all examples of _____.

6a. If you use ICF to code for the fact that *her employer refuses to let her return to work because he feels she is exaggerating the amount of shoulder pain she experiences,* in what domain would you find the code? _____

6b. What letter would represent this domain in the code? _____

7. *Her work station is currently too high for her to reach without shoulder pain.* This italicized phrase is an example of a(n) _____.

8. Sophia would like her employer to agree *to reconfigure her work station by lowering it.* The italicized phrase would be an example of a(n) _____.

9. If you were to use ICF to code her ability *to reach objects on the shelves of her kitchen cabinets,* what type of qualifier would you use? _____

10. If you were to use ICF to code *her ability to reach objects on the shelves of your clinic,* what type of qualifier would you use? _____

11. *Loss of power in all of the abductor and lateral rotator muscles of the glenohumeral joint, a partial tear of the supraspinatus tendon, difficulty combing her hair* and *washing her windows* are all examples of _____ .

12. The *impingement syndrome of her rotator cuff,* and *inflammation in her supraspinatus tendon* both represent what factors in the ICF framework? _____

A Answers to Worksheets

*P*lease note that you should not use Appendix A unless you have already completed the worksheets. Using these pages to initially complete the worksheets deprives the learner of the maximum benefit of this book.

Chapter 3

Medical Terminology: Worksheet 1
Part I
1. Osteoma
2. Hypoglycemia
3. Subcutaneous
4. Suprapubic
5. Dorsal/posterior
6. Cephalad
7. Erythema
8. Intercostal
9. Anterior or ventral
10. Afferent

Part II
1. Fusion of the pubic bones medially (growth of the bones together)
2. Enlargement of the heart
3. Removal of a meniscus
4. Cartilaginous tumor
5. Fusion of a joint
6. Surgical opening of the skull
7. The study of the nervous system
8. Without sensation
9. Inflammation of a vein
10. Abnormally high blood pressure

Medical Terminology: Worksheet 2
Part I
1. Arthritis
2. Arthroscopy
3. Myopathy
4. Dyspnea
5. Ataxia
6. Chondromalacia
7. Encephalitis
8. Meningioma
9. Hemiplegia
10. Subclavicular

Part II
1. Without pain
2. Affecting both sides
3. Opposite side
4. Lack of speech
5. Inflammation of a tendon
6. Slowness of movement
7. Difficulty swallowing
8. Pain in the joints
9. Softening of the brain
10. Pertaining to a rib and its cartilage

Chapter 4

Using Abbreviations: Worksheet 1
1. The physician's orders say to go to physical therapy in a wheelchair and turn the patient every hour.
2. In the medical record it says the diagnosis is rheumatoid arthritis and rule out systemic lupus erythematosus.
3. Intervention Plan: OD, ADL training, US at 1.0 to 1.5 W/cm² to ant sup Ⓡ knee for 5 min.
4. Complains of shortness of breath after bilateral upper extremity proprioceptive neuromuscular facilitation exercises.
5. The medical diagnosis is multiple sclerosis and rule out organic brain syndrome.
6. Pt. has a B/K amputation. Hx of wearing PTB prosthesis c̄ a SACH foot for 20 yrs.
7. Pt. HR ↑ 20 BPM p̄ 2 min. of self-care ADL.
8. Pt amb in parallel bars FWB Ⓛ LE ≈20 ft. ×2 c̄ min. assist. +1. (or min. assist. of 1) for balance
9. UE strength is 5/5 throughout bilat.
10. Anticipated Goal: ↓ dependence in transfers w/c↔bed to mod. assist. within 1 wk.

Using Abbreviations: Worksheet 2
1. The patient complains of right hip pain after ambulating 300 feet once with a walker full weight bearing right lower extremity with minimal assistance of 1 person for balance.
2. Pt. may be 50% PWB Ⓛ LE.
   v.o. Dr. Smith/[your name], PT or OTR
3. Discontinue ultrasound in the area of the right sacroiliac joint.
4. The medical diagnosis is fractured left clavicle and subluxation of the left sternoclavicular joint.

5. Fasting blood sugar upon admission was over 300.
6. Medical dx: CRF.
7. Strength: 4/5 throughout UE bilat.
8. X-ray: fx Ⓛ 3rd metacarpal proximal to MCP joint.
9. To OT for ADL.
   v.o. Dr. Jones/[your name], PT
10. Impression: peripheral neuropathy and rule out central nervous system dysfunction.

Chapter 5

Writing History: Worksheet 1
Part I
1.
2.
3. Hx
4.
5. Hx
6. Hx
7.
8.
9.
10. Hx
11.
12. Hx
13. Hx
14. Hx
15.

Part II
A. 10, 17, 14, 5, 12, 22
B. 3, 27, 13, 15, 30, 19
C. 19
D. 31
E. 20
F. 23, 24, 28, 26
G. 7, 30
H. 1
I. 21, 2
J. 29
K. 16
L. 8, 18, 9, 6, 11
M. 25
N. 4

Part III
1a. Demographics:
1b. Pt. is 83 y.o. African American & is Ⓡ-handed.
2a. Current Condition:
2b. Pt. fell & hit Ⓡ UE & head as she stood up from sofa.
3a. Other clinical tests:
3b. X-ray Ⓡ UE was neg.
4a. Living Environment:
4b. Pt. lives in an assisted living apartment. Meals, laundry, & housekeeping services are provided. Assist c̄ bathing is available prn.

5a. Social Hx:
5b. Pt. stated health care is "unneeded & usually dangerous."

Part IV
Demographics: Pt. is 98 y.o. caucasian ♀ referred by nursing staff & Dr. Frien. Current Condition(s)/Chief Complaint(s): States quit ambulating 10 days ago 2° urinary incontinence c̄ standing. States does not know if she can amb. s̄ urinary incontinence. States keeps a towel in w/c to guard against problems with incontinence. Has not told the nurses & has not seen MD for urinary problem because "women are not supposed to talk with men about those things." States has not yet had any type of Rx for incontinence. States goes to the bathroom frequently to urinate. Pt goals: to be able to amb. to recreational therapy dept. s̄ urinary incontinence problem. Prior Level of Function: Until 1 mo. ago, Pt. was very active in recreational & social activities within the nursing home environment. Social Hx: Pt's family provides emotional support through frequent visits. Employment: Pt. is retired. Living Environment: Has used w/c past 10 days in the nursing home. States transfers in/out of w/c indep. but cannot propel w/c as far as the recreational therapy dept. Social/Health Habits: Pt. does not smoke or drink. Family Hx: htn. Medical/Surgical Hx: Includes htn controlled by medication. Has had difficulties c̄ bladder control for ~5 yrs. & incontinence has ↑ in past few wks. Hx of arthritis in knees for greater than 50 yrs. Functional Status/Activity Level: Pt. stopped amb. during past 2 wks. Currently refuses to amb. c̄ nursing staff. Denies arthritis as cause of refusing to amb. Medications: antihypertensive only. Other Clinical Tests: Urinalysis: normal 1 wk. ago.

Writing History: Worksheet 2
Part I
A. 12, 1
B. 7
C. 30, 21
D. 4
E. 8, 11, 16, 23, 27
F. 22, 10, 26
G. 25, 5, 19
H. 17, 2
I. 20, 28
J. 9, 15 or 15, 9
K. 24, 3
L. 29, 6
M. 14, 18
N. 13

Part II
1.
2.
3.

4. Hx
5. Hx
6.
7. Hx
8.
9. Hx
10.
11. Hx
12.
13. Hx
14.
15.
16. Hx
17.
18. Hx
19.
20.

Part III
1. F
2. B
3. J
4. D
5. N
6. F or I
7. A
8. G
9. A or K
10. E
11. L
12. A
13. G
14. O
15. B
16. J
17. E
18. H
19. A
20. I
21. K
22. A
23. E
24. J
25. A
26. E
27. F
28. O
29. M
30. C

Part IV
Note: Use of brackets [ ] indicates that the statement could have been included in this section of the note or could be where it is listed elsewhere in the note.

HISTORY: <u>Demographics</u>: Pt. is 13 y.o. Caucasian female referred by Dr. Frume c̄ medical dx of subcapital fx ®ᵢₙ hip. [Pt. is ®-handed.] <u>Current condition</u>: c/o "excruciating pain" in ® hip when moves ® LE. Pt. was playing volleyball & jumped & landed on ® hip. <u>Pt. Goals</u>: Pt. wants to return to home ASAP & then to school when she is safe & indep. c̄ ambulation. <u>Prior Level of Function</u>: No prior use of assistive devices. <u>Social Hx</u>: Lives c̄ parents & 11 y.o. brother. Mother does not work outside the home & can assist Pt. upon D/C to home. Pt. has experienced no major life changes during the past year. <u>School</u>: Attends ABC Middle School in 7th grade; school has no steps. <u>Living Environment</u>: Lives in house c̄ carpeted floor surfaces except for kitchen. House has 3 steps to enter c̄ handrail ® ascending. <u>General Health Status</u>: Pt. & mother rate Pt's general health as excellent. <u>Social Health Habits</u>: Denies hx of alcohol or tobacco use. Pt. is on volleyball team & practices volleyball daily. <u>Family Hx</u>: Pt.'s mother has hx of breast CA & ® mastectomy in 1997 c̄ no evidence of recurrence. Father has hx of Htn controlled by medication. Hx of heart disease in maternal & paternal grandfathers. <u>Development</u>: Hx is WNL. Pt. is ®-handed. Pt. <u>Medical/Surgical Hx</u>: No previous injuries or hospitalizations. <u>Functional Status</u>: Pt. has not been out of bed. <u>Medications</u>: Demerol for pain. <u>Other Tests</u>: X-ray shows subcapital fx ® hip c̄ pin in place. Hgb is 10.

Chapter 6

Systems Review: Worksheet 1
Part I
1. SR
2. SR
3. Hx
4. Hx
5. SR
6.
7. SR
8. SR
9. Hx
10. SR
11. Hx
12. Hx
13. SR
14.
15. SR
16. SR
17.
18. Hx
19. SR
20. SR

Part II
1. H
2. C

3. C
4. B
5. F
6. D
7. B
8. A
9. A
10. D
11. C
12. C
13. C
14. J
15. I
16. B
17. A
18. E
19. D
20. G

Part III

SYSTEMS REVIEW: <u>Cardiovascular/Pulmonary System</u>: HR 92 bpm. BP 130/83. RR 30 breaths/min. <u>Integumentary System</u>: Skin integrity: multiple small tears in skin of bilat. UEs noted. Skin texture thin & fragile. Skin color: multiple small hematomas noted below the skin. <u>Musculoskeletal System</u>: Gross AROM: impaired in (R) UE; otherwise WNL. Gross strength: impaired in (R) UE; otherwise unimpaired. Posture: impaired. Ht: 6 ft. 2 in. Wt: 180 lbs. <u>Neuromuscular System</u>: Gait impaired. Locomotion impaired. Balance: impaired. <u>Communication</u>: age-appropriate. <u>Cognition</u>: Oriented to person & place but not to date. <u>Affect</u>: Emotional/behavioral responses impaired when breathing is more difficult. <u>Learning Barriers</u>: requires hearing aid to be able to learn & communicate. <u>Learning Style</u>: best learns from demonstration followed by reminders in the form of pictures. <u>Education needs</u>: disease process, value of exercise, safety, use of adaptive equipment & assist. devices.

Systems Review: Worksheet 2

Part I
1. Hx
2. SR
3. Hx
4. SR
5. Hx
6. SR
7. Hx
8. SR
9. Hx
10. Hx
11. SR
12. Hx
13. SR
14. Hx
15. SR
16. Hx
17. SR
18. Hx
19. SR
20. Hx
21. Hx
22. SR
23. Hx

Part II
1. Cardiovascular/Pulmonary System
2. Cardiovascular/Pulmonary System
3. Musculoskeletal System
4. Musculoskeletal System
5. Musculoskeletal System
6. Integumentary System
7. Integumentary System
8. Neuromuscular System
9. Cardiovascular/Pulmonary System
10. Communication
11. Integumentary System
12. Musculoskeletal System
13. Integumentary System
14. Musculoskeletal System
15. Cognition
16. Education Needs
17. Neuromuscular System
18. Learning Style
19. Learning Barriers
20. Neuromuscular System
21. Affect
22. Cardiovascular/Pulmonary System

Part III

SYSTEMS REVIEW: <u>Cardiovascular/Pulmonary System</u>: Unimpaired. BP: 125/85. HR: 80 bpm. RR: 13 breaths/min. Edema (R) foot surrounding wound on plantar surface. <u>Integumentary System</u>: Impaired. Skin integrity: impaired. Wound noted plantar surface (R) foot. Skin color: red in area surrounding wound. Skin texture: thin & fragile on feet bilaterally. Scar tissue: none noted bilat. <u>Musculoskeletal System</u>: Gross symmetry: impaired LEs. Gross ROM: impaired bilat. feet & ankles. Gross strength: impaired bilat. LEs. Ht. 6 ft. 2 in. Wt. 190 lbs. <u>Neuromuscular System</u>: Locomotion: unimpaired. Gait: impaired. Balance: impaired. <u>Communication</u>: unimpaired. <u>Cognition</u>: orientation unimpaired. <u>Affect</u>: emotional/behavior responses unimpaired. <u>Learning Barriers</u>: Sight impaired 2° cataracts; does not wear glasses. <u>Learning Style</u>: Learns best by demonstration by therapists accompanied by home exercise program that includes illustrations. <u>Education Needs</u>: disease process, safety, wound care, exercise program, ADLs, use of assist. device, general foot care, appropriate foot wear.

Chapter 7

Tests and Measures: Worksheet 1
Part I
 1. TM
 2. Hx
 3.
 4.
 5.
 6. TM
 7. SR
 8. Hx
 9. TM
 10. Hx
 11.
 12. Hx
 13. TM
 14. Hx
 15. TM
 16.
 17.
 18. TM
 19.
 20. Hx

Parts II and III
 1. D
    Impair
 2. B
    Func
 3. E
    Impair
 4. D
    Impair
 5. E
    Impair
 6. E
    Impair
 7. C
    Impair
 8. E
    Impair
 9. E
    Impair
 10. A
    Func
 11. D
    Impair
 12. E
    Impair
 13. B
    Func
 14. D
    Impair
 15. E
    Impair

Part IV
Headings should be the following:
Transfers
Ambulation
Activity Tolerance
Strength
AROM

Part V
A. 2
B. 1
C. 6
D. 4, 3 (any order of these two statements is OK)
E. 5

Part VI
<u>Amb:</u> Pt. stood in parallel bars c̄ min. +1 assist. FWB bilat. LEs 1 min. ×2. Took 1 step c̄ min. +1. <u>Transfers:</u> sit↔stand c̄ min. +1 assist. <u>Activity tolerance:</u> fatigued p̄ standing ×2; all other examination deferred due to fatigue. <u>Strength:</u> UE & LE strength at least 3/5 (group muscle test); unable to further examine due to Pt.'s mental status. <u>ROM:</u> UE & LE WNL except 90° shoulder abduction & 110° shoulder flexion bilat.

Tests and Measures: Worksheet 2
Part I
A. 3, 7
B. 5, 4, 1, 2
C. 6

Part II
There are probably many correct ways to organize this information. This student did a nice job organizing the information. Another way to organize it would be to use the following categories: <u>Amb</u>, <u>Transfers</u>, Ⓡ UE, Ⓛ UE & LEs. This method would allow the reader to see that the Ⓛ UE and LEs are relatively normal and then to get an accurate view of the Ⓡ UE.

TESTS & MEASURES: <u>Amb:</u> c̄ walker c̄ min +1 assist. for 50 ft. ×1 wt. bearing as tolerated all extremities. <u>Transfers:</u> W/c↔mat pivot c̄ min + 1 assist. (or +1 min. assist. or c̄ min. assist. of 1), sit↔supine indep. Ⓡ UE: Appearance: Incision Ⓡ ant. forearm covered c̄ steristrips. AROM: Limited shoulder flex. to 120°, abduction to 70°; elbow flex. WNL, ext. −42°; wrist flex. WNL, ext. to neutral c̄ full finger flex. Strength (gross break test used): shoulder flex. 3+/5; shoulder abduction 3+/5, elbow flex. & ext., wrist flex. & ext., and finger flex. & ext. 4/5. Sensation: WNL to light touch & sharp/dull. Ⓛ UE & LEs: AROM WNL throughout. Strength (gross break test used): 5/5 throughout Ⓛ UE & Ⓡ LE; Ⓛ LE 4/5 all muscle groups. Sensation to light touch & sharp/dull WNL throughout.

Review Worksheet: Writing the History, Systems Review, and Tests and Measures

Part I

1. TM
2.
3.
4. Hx
5. TM
6. Hx
7. Hx
8. Hx
9. TM
10. Hx
11. TM
12. TM
13. Hx
14.
15.

Part II

1a. Hx
1b. Current Condition/chief complaint
1c. C/o intermittent (L) lat. knee pain
2a. Tests and Measures
2b. Sensation
2c. ↓ sensation (L) L5 dermatome
3a. Hx
3b. Other tests
3c. Arthroscopy on 02/02/2002
4a. Hx
4b. Current condition
4c. Craniotomy Feb. 2008
5a. Tests & Measures
5b. PROM
5c. (R) LE PROM is WNL throughout.

Part III

Information in brackets [ ] could go in this category instead of the one in which it was placed.

01/14/2008. HISTORY. <u>Demographic Info.</u>: Pt. is a 65 y.o male patient referred by Dr. Sosome. Medical Dx: fx (R) femoral neck on 01/12/2008. (R) hip prosthesis insertion on 01/13/2008. PT [OT] attempted to see Pt. on 01/14/2008; examination deferred due to low HgB & Pt. dizziness while supine. <u>Current condition</u>: c/o pain (R) hip 8/10 standing & 4/10 supine (prior to amb.). Pt. fell at home & hit (R) hip on bathtub, causing fx. <u>Pt. goals</u>: to amb. indep. s̄ device (long term). [OT: Would like to be indep in grooming & dressing & would "settle" for Meals on Wheels.] Would like to return to her apartment at D/C (short term). <u>Functional status/activity level</u>: States has had no PT or OT PTA. Never used an assist. device PTA. Owns no assist. devices for dressing, grooming, bathing, toileting or amb. PTA watched her toddler-aged grandchildren 1×/wk. <u>Social hx</u>: For recreation PTA watched her toddler-aged grandchildren 1x/wk & played cards c̄ friends 2 noc/wk. <u>Living environment</u>: Lives alone. Lives in a senior apartment building. Has an elevator; has to amb. curbs only. Apartment bathroom has a bathtub c̄ a shower & shower curtain. <u>Employment status</u>: Retired in past yr from teaching. Volunteers at elementary school 3 days/wk., reading c̄ children. <u>Social/health habits</u>: denies ETOH use & does not smoke. Walks ~2 mi. 3×/wk. <u>Medical/surgical hx</u>: Pt. took no medications PTA. Describes herself as healthy. <u>Other clinical tests</u>: HgB 7 on 01/14/2008. Received blood transfusion on 01/14/2008. HbG 11 on this date.

SYSTEMS REVIEW. <u>Cardiopulmonary</u>: unimpaired. BP 140/80. HR 80 bpm. Resp. rate 12 breaths/min. <u>Integumentary</u>: impaired at surgery site; otherwise unimpaired. <u>Musculoskeletal</u>: Gross strength impaired (R) LE. Gross ROM impaired (R) LE. <u>Neuromuscular system</u>: gait impaired, locomotion impaired, balance impaired in standing & during amb., motor function impaired. Communication: unimpaired. <u>Affect</u>: emotional/behavioral responses unimpaired. <u>Cognition</u>: oriented ×3. Unimpaired. <u>Learning barriers</u>: wears glasses & cannot read s̄ them; will need glasses to learn home exercise program. <u>Learning style</u>: visual learner; prefers to watch & then imitate PT's actions. <u>Education needs</u>: amb. training & safety c̄ walker on level surfaces & curbs, transfer training & safety, info. on proper progression & healing of incision site, home exercise program. —————

TESTS & MEASURES [PT]: <u>Transfers</u>: w/c↔bed & supine↔sit c̄ mod. + 1 assist. Sit↔stand c̄ min. +1 assist. <u>Amb.</u>: in parallel bars ~20 ft. ×1 50% PWB (R) LE c̄ min. + 1 assist. Pt. became dizzy & nauseated p̄ amb. & further examination & interventions during this PT session terminated p̄ amb. Nurses notified of nausea. <u>Exercise tolerance</u>: BP 145/90 p amb., 135/80 3 min. p̄ amb. HR 105 bpm p̄ amb., 82 bpm 3 min. p̄ amb. Resp Rate: 18 p̄ amb., 12 3 min. p̄ amb. <u>UEs & (L) LE</u>: Strength 4+/5 throughout per group muscle test. ROM: WNL except −5° (R) elbow ext. (R) <u>LE</u>: ROM: limited 2° post-op restrictions to 90° hip flex, full active hip abduction, 0° hip medial & lateral rotation, 0° adduction. Strength: at least 3/5 throughout per group muscle tests; not further examined 2° recent surgery. —————

TESTS & MEASURES (OT). Pt. initially seen B/S for examination of grooming & dressing skills. <u>Bathing</u>: Able to bathe UEs & trunk c̄ supervision & setup of sponge bath; requires min. +1 assist. to bathe LEs. <u>Grooming</u>: Grooms hair indep. Dental care indep. Contact lens management indep. <u>Dressing</u>: not tested this date 2° high pain level & ↓ Pt. endurance. <u>Transfers</u>: supine↔sit & w/c↔bed c̄ mod. assist. of 1. <u>UEs</u>: Strength 4+/5 per group muscle test. AROM: WNL except −5° (R) elbow ext. Fine motor skills WNL. Currently has IV infusing in (L) forearm. —————

Chapter 9

Subjective: Worksheet 1
Part I
1. S
2.
3. [This is not S because the results of tests and measures are required to ascertain whether the motion reproduces the pain.]
4.
5.
6. S
7.
8.
9. S
10. Prob
11.
12.
13.
14. S
15.
16. Prob
17.
18.
19.
20. S
21.
22. S

Part II
1. Dx: Ⓡ shoulder bursitis.
2. Problem: 75 y.o. caucasian ♂ c̄ dx of Ⓛ shoulder subluxation. S/p Ⓡ-side stroke Ⓛ hemiparesis ~1 yr.
3. Dx: respiratory failure. Hx: COPD, CHF, Htn

Part III
A. Current condition: 1, 4, 6, 2, 12
B. Prior level of function: 8, 9
C. Patient goals: 10, 7
D. Social history: 3, 17, 21, [19 could go here but is better placed with statement about the patient's ability to garden]
E. Employment status: 16
F. Living environment: 22
G. General health status: 11
H. Social/health habits: 24
I. Family/health history: 14
J. Functional status/activity level: 5, 18, 19, 20
K. Medical/surgical history: 8, 13
L. Medications: 23

Part IV
1a. Current condition:
1b. Pt. fell in her living room.
1c. (1) When did the patient fall?
   (2) How did the patient fall?
   (3) What was the patient doing when she fell?
2a. Current condition:
2b. States onset of pain in the p.m. of [date].
3a. Current condition:
3b. C/o pain Ⓡ foot on this date.
3c. (1) The exact location of the pain in the Ⓡ foot.
   (2) Rating the pain on a pain scale.
4a. Living environment:
4b. States lives alone. Describes 2 steps c̄ handrail on Ⓡ ascending at entrance of her home.
5a. Current condition:
5b. States pain radiates from Ⓡ hand through Ⓡ forearm on this date, limiting typing to 5 min. ā requires rest.

Part V
Problem: 58 y.o. ♂ referred from E.D. by Dr. Othrop. Medical dx: minor ligamentous injury Ⓡ knee. X-ray Ⓡ knee negative. —————————
   S: <u>Current Condition:</u> c/o constant, "burning" Ⓡ knee pain; rates pain as 7 (0 = no pain, 10 = worst possible pain). Pain ↓ c̄ rest & ↑ c̄ walking. Denies pain while bending Ⓡ knee. Fell at work & landed on Ⓡ knee. <u>Prior level of function:</u> Denies former difficulty with amb. Denies previous use of crutches. <u>Patient goals:</u> Short term: to be able to access apartment indep. Long term: to resume former busy lifestyle, including returning to work asap. <u>Social history:</u> Lives c̄ wife; wife works & is not available to assist. Pt. during the day. Employment status: States is a carpenter; is on his feet most of the work day. <u>Living environment:</u> Lives in apartment on 2nd floor c̄ 9 steps to enter c̄ handrail on the Ⓛ ascending. No elevator is available. <u>General health status:</u> States general health is good. <u>Social/health habits:</u> gets lots of exercise each day at work. Does not smoke. <u>Family health history:</u> Htn in 2/5 siblings & both parents. <u>Functional status:</u> Is having difficult amb. States can borrow crutches from a co-worker. <u>Medical/Surgical History:</u> No significant history of disease, serious illness, or injury. History of spring allergies. <u>Medications:</u> Takes [prescription allergy medication]. —————————
Progress note follows:
   S: <u>Current condition:</u> c/o pain c̄ typing; rates pain as 5 (0 = no pain, 10 = worst pain). Pain ↓ c̄ rest & ↑ c̄ grasping or wt. bearing activities Ⓛ UE. Fell at work [date] & landed on Ⓛ hand c̄ wrist extended so pain has ↑ since last seen by PT on [date]. States x-rays of Ⓛ wrist & hand at physician's office p̄ fall were neg. Also c/o edema & stiffness Ⓛ hand & wrist c̄ active movement. Edema is ↑ p̄ work. <u>New Pt. goal:</u> to be able to hold a fork s̄ pain (short term). <u>Employment:</u> Pt. types at work up to 8 hrs./day. States physician told him to limit typing to 4 hrs./day until edema stops. <u>Functional activities:</u> is having difficulty eating c̄ Ⓡ hand; is Ⓛ hand dominant. —————————

Subjective: Worksheet 2

Part I

A. Current condition: 9, 1
B. Prior level of function: 7
C. Pt. goals: 10, 2
D. Social hx: 4
E. Employment status: 11
F. Living environment: 3, 5
G. General health status: 13
H. Social/health habits: 14
I. Family health hx: 12
J. Functional status: 7
K. Medical/surgical hx: 6, 8
L. Medications: 15

Part II

1a. Current condition
1b. C/o pain (R) LE proximal to the knee.
1c. (1) Exact location of the pain is still unclear. Is the pain in the anterior or posterior portion of the (R) LE proximal to the knee?
(2) Putting the pain on a pain scale would have been helpful.
2a. Prior level of function/social history (either answer would be correct)
2b. States depended on his wife to bathe him prior to this stroke. Plans to cont. to depend on wife for bathing p̄ D/C.
3a. Functional activities
3b. States cannot dress herself.
4a. Functional activities
4b. Denies use of a walker PTA.

Part III

1.
2.
3.
4. S
5.
6.
7. S
8.
9.
10. Prob
11. S
12.
13.
14.
15. S
16.
17.
18.
19. S

Part IV

Problem: Pt. is 65 y.o. ♀ Pt. of Dr. Grimee. Medical dx: Contusion (L) hip.

S: Current condition: C/o (L) hip pain when FWB (L) LE; pain intensity is 8 (0 = no pain; 10 = worst possible pain). Denies pain when in sitting or supine position. Fell on (L) hip at home in morning; was able to get up s̄ help. States experienced pain throughout day & went to ED in late p.m. Prior level of function: Amb. indep. s̄ assist. device & all ADL tasks indep. prior to injury. Pt. goals: To indep. perform all ADL tasks s̄ walker. Social history: Types bulletin & helps clean at her church on a volunteer basis. Lives alone; husband died 10 years ago. Employment status: Pt. is retired. Living environment: Lives in apartment c̄ an elevator. Needs to amb. curbs only. General health status: States she is in good health. Social/health habits: Does not smoke or drink ETOH. Family health history: Both parents are living. Mother has osteoporosis. Current functional ability: Currently spends time in a w/c rented by the family. Medical/surgical history: unremarkable except total hip replacement (L) in 2000; used a walker at that time. No history of hospitalization except for childbearing. Medications: Does not take medications.

Chapter 10

Objective: Worksheet 1

Part I

1.
2. O
3.
4. S
5. O
6. S
7.
8. S
9. Prob
10. O
11.
12. O
13. S
14.
15. S
16.
17.
18.
19. O
20. O
21.
22. S
23.

Part II

1. B
2. B
3. B
4. A

5. B
6. B
7. A
8. B
9. B
10. B
11. B
12. B
13. A
14. B

Part III

1a. Strength
1b. Pt. has 4/5 strength in bilat. UEs.
2a. Trunk
2b. SLR Ⓛ LE reproduces Pt.'s worst back pain.
3a. Strength
3b. 5/5 Ⓡ shoulder musculature, 4/5 Ⓡ biceps, 2/5 Ⓡ triceps, 0/5 Ⓡ UE musculature distal to elbow. Ⓛ UE musculature is 5/5.
4a. Amb.
4b. Pt. amb. ~150 ft. FWB c̄ walker ×2 indep.
5a. Reaction to Rx:
5b. Pt. was SOB p̄ transfers supine↔sit and bed↔B/S chair; resp. rate ↑ from 18 breaths/min. ā transfer to 32 breaths/min. immediately p̄ the transfer.
6a. AROM
6b. Ⓛ ankle is WNL.

Part IV

1. Cardiovascular: unimpaired. BP 110/65. HR 75 bpm. Resp. rate 14 breaths/min.
2. Integumentary: unimpaired.
3. Musculoskeletal: impaired Ⓡ LE.
4. Neuromuscular: impaired gait & locomotion; motor function unimpaired; balance impaired.
5. Communication: age-appropriate & unimpaired.
6. Affect: unimpaired.
7. Cognition: unimpaired; oriented ×3.
8. Learning barriers: none noted.
9. Learning style: visual; prefers demonstration prior to attempting movement.
10. Educational needs: amb. c̄ walker & walker safety; transfer safety; protection of cast
11. Bilat UEs: Strength & AROM WNL.
12. Amb.: indep. c̄ walker NWB Ⓛ LE 50 ft. ×2.
13. Ⓛ LE: long leg cast applied.
14. Ⓡ LE: AROM WNL. Strength 5/5 throughout.
15. Transfers: on/off toilet c̄ min. +1 assist. Sit↔stand & supine↔sit indep.
16. Amb.: ↑ & ↓ 1 step c̄ walker NWB Ⓛ LE c̄ min. +1 assist.
17. Amb.: in & out of door, including opening & closing door, c̄ walker c̄ min. +1 assist.
18. Ⓛ LE: Not examined further this date.
19. Ht. 5'6"; wt. 165 lbs.

Part V

A. Cardiovascular: 1
B. Integumentary: 2
C. Musculoskeletal: 3, 19
D. Neuromuscular: 4
E. Communication: 5
F. Affect: 6
G. Cognition: 7
H. Learning Barriers: 8
I. Learning Style: 9
J. Ed. Needs: 10
K. Amb: 12, 17, 16
L. Transfers: 15
M. UEs & Ⓡ LE: 11, 14
N. Ⓛ LE: 13, 18

Part VI

O: SYSTEMS REVIEW: Cardiovascular: unimpaired. BP 110/65. HR 75 bpm. Resp. rate 14 breaths/min. Integumentary: unimpaired. Musculoskeletal: impaired Ⓡ LE. Ht. 5'6"; wt. 165 lbs. Neuromuscular: impaired gait & locomotion, motor function unimpaired, balance impaired. Communication: age-appropriate & unimpaired. Affect: unimpaired. Cognition: unimpaired; oriented ×3. Learning barriers: none noted. Learning style: visual; prefers demonstration prior to attempting movement. Educational needs: amb. c̄ walker & walker safety; transfer safety; protection of cast. TESTS & MEASURES: Amb: Indep. c̄ walker NWB Ⓛ LE 50 ft. ×2. Amb. ↑ & ↓ 1 step & in/out of door, including opening & closing door, c̄ walker NWB Ⓛ LE c̄ min. + 1 assist. Transfers: On/off toilet c̄ min. + 1 assist. Sit↔stand & supine↔sit indep. UEs & Ⓡ LE: Strength & AROM WNL throughout. Ⓛ LE: long let cast applied. Not examined further this date.——————

Objective: Worksheet 2

Part I

A. 6
B. 1
C. 2
D. 7, 4, 3, 5

Part II

O: TESTS & MEASUREMENTS: W/c propulsion & management: Propels w/c indep. 15 ft. ×1. Has difficulty parking w/c close to mat & locking brakes. Requires max +1 assist to remove armrest. Transfers: w/c↔mat c̄ sliding board NWB Ⓡ LE c̄ min +1 assist.to maintain NWB Ⓡ LE & verbal cues for hand placement; requires max +1 assist. to place sliding board. Sit↔supine c̄ mod. +1 assist to move Ⓡ LE. LE Strength: Hip flexors: 4/5 Ⓛ, 3−/5 Ⓡ. Hip extensors: 4/5 Ⓛ, 3/5 Ⓡ. Hip abduction bilat. at least 3/5; not tested c̄ resistance against gravity due to patient fatigue. Knee flexors: 4/5 Ⓛ; 2−/5 Ⓡ. Knee extensors: 4/5 Ⓛ; 3/5 Ⓡ. Ankle 5/5 strength bilat.

all movements. <u>Reaction to Rx</u>: Performed Ⓡ & Ⓛ hip abd/add. c̄ 2# ×15 repetitions (supine); knee flex. c̄ 2# ×15 repetitions Ⓛ, 1# ×15 repetitions Ⓡ; bilat. terminal knee ext. c̄ 2# ×15 rep. Requires frequent rests during exercise; activity tolerance & muscle endurance are low.

PART III

1a. TESTS & MEASURES, Ambulation or Gait subsection
1b. Amb. c̄ walker 50% PWB Ⓛ LE for 50 ft. ×2 c̄ verbal cues to compensate for vision deficits.
2a. SYSTEMS REVIEW; Cardiopulmonary subsection.
2b. Pitting edema Ⓛ LE noted.
3a. TESTS & MEASURES, Reflexes subsection
3b. KJ: increased Ⓡ, normal Ⓛ
4a. TESTS & MEASURES, Transfers subsection
4b. Transfers w/c↔mat c̄ min. assist. of 1 to stabilize balance loss.
5a. TESTS & MEASURES, Rolling or Bed Mobility subsection
5b. Requires max assist. of 2 to roll supine→ Ⓡ or Ⓛ.
6a. SYSTEMS REVIEW, Learning Barriers subsection
6b. No learning barriers noted.

Review Worksheet: Stating the Problem, S, and O

Part I
1. O
2.
3.
4. S
5. O
6. Prob, in some facilities, could be in O part of the note
7. S
8. S
9. O
10. Prob
11. O
12. O
13. S
14.
15.

Part II
1a. Subjective, or S
1b. Current condition
1c. C/o intermittent Ⓛ lat. knee pain
2a. Objective, or O
2b. TESTS & MEASURES, Sensation
2c. ↓ sensation Ⓛ L5 dermatome.
3a. Subjective, or S
3b. Current condition
3c. States had an arthroscopy on 02/02/2008
4a. Subjective, or S
4b. Current condition
4c. States had craniotomy in Feb. 2002

5a. Objective, or O
5b. Ⓡ LE or PROM or ROM
5c. Ⓡ LE PROM is WNL throughout

Part III
01/15/2008 PROBLEM: Pt. is a 65 y.o. ♂ Pt. of Dr. Sosome. Medical Dx: Fx Ⓡ femoral neck 01/12/2008. Ⓡ hip prosthesis inserted 01/14/2008. HgB 7 on 01/14/2008. Pt received blood transfusion on 01/14/2008. HgB 11 on this date. PT attempted to see Pt. on 01/14/2008 & did not see Pt. due to HgB of 7 & Pt. c/o dizziness while supine. ——————————————

S: <u>Current condition</u>: c/o pain Ⓡ LE 8/10 (0 = no pain, 10 = worst possible pain) while standing & 4/10 supine (prior to amb.). States fell at home & Ⓡ hip hit side of bathtub. <u>Prior level of function</u>: States was indep. c̄ amb. s̄ assist. devices & all types of ADL activities PTA. Never received PT or OT services PTA. <u>Pt. goals</u>: Would like to return to her apartment p̄ D/C. (PT:) Would like to amb. indep s̄ device (long term). (OT:) Would like to be indep. in grooming & dressing herself; would accept Meals on Wheels. <u>Social hx</u>: Lives alone. <u>Employment status</u>: Retired in past yr. from teaching school. Volunteers at elementary school 3 days/wk., reading c̄ children. For recreation, Pt. plays cards c̄ friends 2 nocs/wk. & watches toddler-aged grandchildren 1x/wk. <u>Living environment</u>: Lives in senior apartment building c̄ elevator; needs to amb. curbs only to enter. Apartment bathroom has bathtub c̄ shower & shower curtain. Owns no assist. devices for bathing, toileting, dressing, or amb. <u>General health status</u>: States she is in good health. <u>Social/health habits</u>: Does not smoke or drink ETOH. Walked ~2 mi. 3×/wk. PTA. <u>Family health hx</u>: Pt.'s parents are alive & in their 90's & in good health. <u>Functional status/activity level</u>: States required the assist. of 2 people to transfer into B/S chair earlier on this date. <u>Medical/surgical hx</u>: Denies previous hospitalizations or fx prior to this date. <u>Medications</u>: States takes no medications at home.

O: SYSTEMS REVIEW: <u>Cardiopulmonary</u>: unimpaired. BP 120/80. HR 80 bpm. Resp. rate 12 breaths/min. <u>Integumentary</u>: impaired at surgery site; otherwise unimpaired. <u>Musculoskeletal</u>: ROM & gross strength impaired on Ⓡ LE. Ht. 5'11"; wt. 170 lbs. <u>Neuromuscular</u>: gait, locomotion, balance in standing & during amb. & motor function impaired. <u>Communication</u>: unimpaired. <u>Affect</u>: emotional/behavioral responses unimpaired. <u>Cognition</u>: oriented ×3, unimpaired. <u>Learning barriers</u>: wears glasses & cannot read s̄ them; will need glasses for home exercise program. <u>Learning style</u>: visual learner; prefers watching therapist & then imitating actions of therapist. <u>Educational needs</u>: use of walker on level surfaces & curbs & safety c̄ walker, transfer training & safety, proper wound healing & monitoring of incision site, home exercise program. TESTS & MEASURES: <u>Transfers</u>: w/c↔bed & supine↔sit c̄ moderate assist. of 1 person. Sit↔stand c̄ min assist. of 1 person. <u>Amb</u>: in parallel bars c̄ min. assist. of 1 person ~20 ft. ×1 PWB Ⓡ LE; Pt. then felt dizzy & nauseated so PT session was terminated at that time & nurses were notified of Pt's nausea. UEs & Ⓛ LE: ROMs WNL throughout except –5° Ⓡ elbow extension. Strength 4+/5 throughout (group muscle test). Ⓡ LE: ROM limited 2° post-op restrictions to 90° hip flex, full hip abduction, 0° hip medial & lateral rotation, 0° adduction. Strength: at least 3/5 throughout; not examined further 2° recent surgery. Exercise tolerance: BP 145/90 immediately p̄ amb, 135/80 3 min. p̄ amb. HR 105 bpm immediately p̄ amb, 82 bpm 3 min. p̄ amb. Resp. rate 18 breaths/min. immediately p̄ amb, 12 breaths/min. 3 min. p̄ amb. ————————————

[For the OT, beginning c̄ the section on transfers:]

Transfers: w/c↔bed & supine↔sit c̄ mod + 1 assist. Bathing: Able to bathe trunk & arms c̄ supervision & setup of sponge bath; bathes LEs c̄ min. +1 assist. Grooming: Grooms hair indep. Dental care indep. Indep. management of contact lenses from w/c. Dressing: not assessed this date 2° ↑ pain level & ↓ Pt. endurance. UEs: Strength 4+/5 throughout (group muscle test). AROMs WNL except –5° Ⓡ elbow extension. Fine motor skills WNL. ————————————

Chapters 11, 12 & 13

Worksheet 1
Part I
1. T & M
2. Systems Review
3. Hx
4. Hx
5. Hx
6.
7. Eval.
8.
9. Prog.
10. Hx
11. Hx
12. Hx
13. Prog.
14. T & M
15. Systems Review
16.
17. Hx
18. Prog.
19. Diag.
20. Prog.
21. Hx
22. T & M

Part II
1. Eval.
2. Prog.
3. Prog.
4. Eval.
5. Prog.

Part III
1. EVALUATION: Gait deviations & need for assist. in amb. c̄ an assist. device prevent Pt. from functioning at home indep. & from doing her work as a cashier outside of the home. Inability to use Ⓛ UE in a functional manner is affecting Pt.'s ability to perform ADLs. ————————————
DIAGNOSIS: Practice Patterns: 1° Neuromuscular D: Impaired Motor Function & Sensory Integrity Associated c̄ Nonprogressive Disorders of the CNS—Acquired in Adolescence or Adulthood. 2° Musculoskeletal G: Impaired Joint Mobility, Muscle Performance, & ROM Associated c̄ Fx. Neuromuscular Pattern is 1° due to greater extent of deficits involved. ————————————
PROGNOSIS: Pt. has good rehabilitation potential. Pt. is relatively young, motivated, cooperative & cognitively sound. ————————————
2. EVALUATION: ↓ function in transfers is impairing Pt.'s ability to participate in activities in nursing home and is placing the health of nursing home staff at risk. ————————————
DIAGNOSIS: Practice Pattern Musculoskeletal J: Impaired Joint Mobility, Motor Function, Muscle Performance & ROM Associated c̄ Amputation. ————————————
PROGNOSIS: Rehabilitation potential is fair because of Pt.'s medical dx of Alzheimer's Disease. Pt. follows simple commands & should be able to learn to transfer bed↔w/c c̄ min. assist. of 1 & verbal cues. This would ↓ risk & burden to caretakers, maximize activity level & quality of life, & prevent further pulmonary & integumentary problems. ————————————

Worksheet 2
Part I
1. S
2.
3. O (SYSTEMS REVIEW)
4. O (TESTS & MEASURES)
5. O (TESTS & MEASURES)
6.
7. Diag.
8. S
9. Prob.
10. O (TESTS & MEASURES)
11. Diag.
12. O (SYSTEMS REVIEW)
13. S
14. Prog.
15. Prog.
16. O (TESTS & MEASURES)
17. O (SYSTEMS REVIEW)
18. Diag.

19. O (TESTS & MEASURES)
20. Prog.

Part II
1. Prog.
2. Eval.
3. Diag.
4. Prog.
5. Eval.

Part III
1. EVALUATION: Pt.'s ↓ ROM & strength Ⓡ wrist are associated c̄ Pt. difficulty in ADLS such as eating & writing. Pt.'s work involves typing over 50% of the time & Pt. is unable to type s̄ pain. DIAGNOSIS: Practice Pattern: Musculoskeletal G: Impaired Joint Mobility, Muscle Performance, & ROM Associated c̄ Fx. PROGNOSIS: Pt. has good rehab. potential; should progress well with PT.
2. EVALUATION: Pt.'s Ⓡ extremity strength, motor planning & mobility impairments will prevent the Pt. from returning home alone. Will need to regain indep. amb. & ADLs to return home. DIAGNOSIS: Practice Pattern: Neuromuscular D: Impaired Motor Function & Sensory Integrity Associated c̄ Nonprogressive Disorders of the CNS—Acquired in Adolescence or Adulthood. PROGNOSIS: Rehab. potential is fair. Pt. may need prolonged time to regain movement of Ⓛ extremities & overall mobility due to her advanced age.

Review Worksheet: History, Systems Review, Tests & Measures, Diagnosis, Prognosis/ Problem, S, O, A

PART I. History, Systems Review, Tests & Measures, Diagnosis, Prognosis

HISTORY: <u>Demographics</u>: Pt. is a 65 y.o. ♂ c̄ a dx of DJD Ⓡ hip c a THA on [date]. Physician is Dr. Sienn. Pt. is Ⓡ-hand dominant. <u>Current Condition</u>: c/o Ⓡ hip pain in area of sutures of the following intensities: 7 when moving, 3 when sitting, 2 when lying still (0 = no pain, 10 = worst possible pain). Does not recall precautions for Pts. c̄ THA. PTA pain was constant & intensity was 9 or 10. <u>Pt. goals</u>: Pt. wants to eventually return to gardening & yard work activities. <u>Prior Level of Function</u>: Immediately PTA, Pt. amb. s̄ assist. device. PTA attempted amb. for exercise daily; was only able to amb. 1 block PTA. Two yrs. ago Pt. was able to amb. 1 mi. or more. <u>Social Hx</u>: Lives c̄ his wife in his own home. Plans to return home c̄ his wife p̄ D/C. <u>Employment</u>: Pt. is retired. <u>Living Environment</u>: Has 1 step to enter home c̄ railing on Ⓡ ascending. Owns a 3-in-1 commode, a walker, & a cane. <u>General Health Status</u>: Pt. rates general health as good; no major life changes in past yr. <u>Social/Health Habits</u>: Does not smoke; only occasionally drinks ETOH. <u>Family Hx</u>: Pt.'s father died of MI at age

78. Pt.'s mother died of breast CA at age 72. Pt. has no siblings. <u>Medical/Surgical Hx</u>: Hx of htn. Hx of hospitalization for Ⓛ THA on 01/10/2007. <u>Functional Status/ Activity Level</u>: Hobby is gardening. Gardens outside of the church. Does volunteer ushering at church. <u>Medications</u>: Takes [antihypertensive medication]. ————

SYSTEMS REVIEW: <u>Cardiovascular/pulmonary</u>: not impaired. HR 80 bpm. Resp. rate 14 breaths/min. BP 130/85. <u>Edema</u>: none noted. <u>Integumentary</u>: impaired. Disruption: staples Ⓡ hip. Skin color WNL. Skin texture not tested this date. <u>Musculoskeletal</u>: Gross symmetry not impaired. Gross ROM & strength impaired Ⓡ hip & knee. Ht: 6 ft. 0 in. Wt: 185 lbs. <u>Neuromuscular</u>: Gait impaired. <u>Locomotion</u>: impaired transfers & bed mobility. Balance impaired in standing; uses walker. Not impaired in sitting. Motor function not impaired. <u>Communication</u> not impaired. <u>Cognition</u>: oriented ×3; not impaired. <u>Learning barriers</u>: cannot read s̄ glasses. <u>Education needs</u>: home exercise program, precautions for Pts. c̄ THA, progression of recovery process, use of walker, ADLs including transfers. <u>Learning style</u>: prefers demonstration ā trying an activity; visual learner. ————

TESTS & MEASURES: <u>Amb</u>: Stood B/S c̄ walker 10% PWB Ⓡ LE c̄ mod. assist. of 1 for 1 minute ×2. <u>Transfers</u>: Supine↔sit c̄ min. assist. of 1. Sit↔stand & w/c↔ mat pivot c̄ mod. assist. of 1. Toilet transfers not tested this date. Ⓡ LE: Strength grossly 1/5 in hip & knee musculature; ankle dorsiflexion 4+/5; ankle plantar flexion at least 2/5 but not tested further due to 10% PWB status. PROM: 0–20° hip flexion, 0–10° hip abduction, 0° hip extension; adduction, medial & lateral rotation of hip not tested due to hip precautions & recent surgery. Knee flexion: 0–70°. AROM: Ⓡ ankle WNL. Incision Ⓡ hip 10 cm long over greater trochanter; staples intact. UE & Ⓛ LE: AROM WNL & strength 4+/5 throughout bilat. UEs & Ⓛ LE. Group muscle testing performed UEs; individual muscle testing performed LEs. ————

EVALUATION: Indep. amb. c̄ a walker is necessary for Pt. to return to home. Impairments of ↓ ROM & strength Ⓡ LE are associated with dependent amb. on this date. ————

DIAGNOSIS: Practice Pattern Musculoskeletal H: Impaired Joint Mobility, Motor Function, Muscle Performance & ROM Associated c̄ Joint Arthroplasty. ————

PROGNOSIS: Pt. has good rehab. potential. His level of function was good PTA & he has a great desire to return to ā healthy, active lifestyle in the community. Should be able to return to home c̄ his wife indep. in amb. & ā home exercise program to cont. to ↑ Ⓡ LE strength & ROM c̄ 2–3 days of therapy BID. ————

PART II. Problem, S, O, and A

Problem: Pt. is a 65 y.o. ♂ c̄ a dx of DJD Ⓡ hip c̄ a THA on [date]. Physician is Dr. Sienn. Hx of hospitalization for Ⓛ THA on 01/10/2007. Hx of htn. Takes [antihypertensive medication]. ————————————

S: <u>Current Condition</u>: c/o Ⓡ hip pain in area of sutures of the following intensities: 7 when moving, 3 when sitting, 2 when lying still (0 = no pain, 10 = worst possible pain). PTA pain was constant & intensity was 9 or 10. Does not recall precautions for Pt.'s c̄ THA. <u>Prior Level of Function</u>: Immediately PTA, Pt amb. s̄ assist. device. PTA attempted amb. for exercise daily; was only able to amb. 1 block PTA. Two yrs. ago Pt. was able to amb. 1 mi. or more. <u>Pt. Goals</u>: Pt. wants to eventually return to gardening & yard work activities. <u>Social hx</u>: Lives c̄ his wife in his own home. Plans to return home c̄ his wife p̄ D/C. <u>Employment</u>: Pt. is retired. <u>Living Environment</u>: Has 1 step to enter home c̄ railing on Ⓡ ascending. Owns a 3-in-1 commode, a walker, & a cane. <u>General Health Status</u>: Pt. rates general health as good; no major life changes in past yr. <u>Social Health Habits</u>: Does not smoke; only occasionally drinks ETOH. <u>Family Hx</u>: Pt.'s father died of MI at age 78. Pt.'s mother died of breast CA at age 72. Pt. has no siblings. <u>Functional Status/Activity Level</u>: Hobby is gardening. Gardens outside of the church. Does volunteer ushering at church. Pt. is Ⓡ-hand dominant. <u>Medical/Surgical Hx</u>: Hx of htn. Hx of hospitalization for Ⓛ THA on 01/10/2007. <u>Medications</u>: Takes [antihypertensive medication] ————————————

O: SYSTEMS REVIEW: <u>Cardiovascular/pulmonary</u>: not impaired. HR 80 bpm. Resp. rate 14 breaths/min. BP 130/85. Edema: none noted. <u>Integumentary</u>: impaired. Disruption: staples Ⓡ hip. Skin color WNL. Skin texture not tested this date. <u>Musculoskeletal</u>: Gross symmetry not impaired. Gross ROM & strength: impaired Ⓡ hip & knee. Ht: 6 ft. 0 in. Wt: 185 lbs. <u>Neuromuscular</u>: Gait impaired. <u>Locomotion</u>: impaired transfers & bed mobility. Balance impaired in standing; uses walker. Not impaired in sitting. Motor function: not impaired. Communication not impaired. <u>Cognition</u>: oriented ×3; not impaired. <u>Learning barriers</u>: cannot read s̄ glasses. <u>Education needs</u>: home exercise program, precautions for Pts. c̄ THA, progression of recovery process, use of walker, ADLs including transfers. Learning style: prefers demonstration ā trying an activity. TESTS & MEASURES: <u>Amb.</u>: Stood B/S c̄ walker 10% PWB Ⓡ LE c̄ mod. assist. of 1 for 1 minute ×2. <u>Transfers</u>: Supine↔sit c̄ min. assist of 1. Sit↔stand & w/c↔mat pivot c̄ mod. assist. of 1. Toilet transfers not tested this date due to decreased activity tolerance of Pt. this date. Ⓡ LE: Strength grossly 1/5 in hip & knee musculature; ankle dorsiflexion 4+/5; ankle plantar flexion at least 2/5 but not tested further due to 10% PWB status. PROM: 0–20° hip flexion, 0–10° hip abduction, 0° hip extension; adduction, medical & lateral rotation of hip not tested due to hip precautions & recent surgery. Knee flexion: 0–70°. AROM: Ⓡ ankle WNL. Incision Ⓡ hip 0 cm long over greater trochanter; staples intact. UE & Ⓛ LE: AROM WNL & strength 4+/5 throughout bilat. UEs & Ⓛ LE group muscle testing performed UEs; individual muscle testing performed LEs. ————————————

A: EVALUATION: Indep. amb. c̄ a walker is necessary for Pt. to return to home. Impairments of ↓ ROM & strength Ⓡ LE are associated c̄ dependent amb. on this date. DIAGNOSIS: Practice Pattern Musculoskeletal H: Impaired Joint Mobility, Motor Function, Muscle Performance & ROM Associated c̄ Joint Arthroplasty. PROGNOSIS: Pt. has good rehab. potential. His level of function was good PTA & he has a great desire to return to a healthy, active lifestyle in the community. Should be able to return to home c̄ his wife indep. in amb. & a home exercise program to cont. to ↑ Ⓡ LE strength & ROM p̄ 2–3 days of therapy BID. ————————————

Chapter 14:

Writing Expected Outcomes Worksheet 1
Part I
1. A. Pt. (implied)
   B. will manage & propel w/c
   C. a w/c must be present; Pt. must be at home
   D. indep. (observable)
   ~ 50 ft. ×10 (measurable)
   within 1 mo. (time frame)
   to allow Pt. to function at home (functional)
2. A. Pt.
   B. will demonstrate amb.
   C. c̄ prosthesis
   s̄ device
   stairs must be present
   uneven surfaces must be present
   D. on at least 14 stairs (measurable)
   for at least 1/2 mi. on even & uneven surfaces (measurable & observable)
   indep. (observable)
   within 2 wks. (time frame)
   to ensure Pt.'s ability to amb. in & out of his home & around his yard (functional)
3. A. Pt.
   B. will demonstrate body mechanics
   C. while lifting up to 50 lbs.
   D. body mechanics will be good (observable)
   to allow Pt. to return to work fully functional at performing his job (functional)
   within 4 wks. of Rx (time frame)
4. A. Pt.
   B. will demonstrate rolling
   C. Pt. must have a place to roll (implied)
   D. indep. in segmental rolling (observable)
   c̄ 6 mo. of Rx (time frame)
   to make Pt. more functional as she sleeps & plays (functional)

Part II

1. Pt. will amb. c̄ crutches on level surfaces & 1 step elevation 40 ft. ×3 NWB Ⓛ LE indep. p̄ 2 days of Rx to allow Pt. to get around her house for ADL.
2. Pt. will demonstrate care & wrapping of her residual limb c̄ elastic wrap indep. applying even pressure 100% of the time within 3 days to prepare for training in amb. c̄ a prosthesis.
3. Pt. will be able to lift a 5 lb. box from an overhead cupboard & place it on a table using bilat. UEs equally within 2 mo. to enable Pt.'s ability to reach items on the shelves in her kitchen & closet at home during ADL.
4. Pt. will amb. s̄ assist. device in her home for 50 ft. ×4 using pursed lip breathing pattern within 4 wks. of Rx to enable her to cook & perform ADLs.

Part III

1. Pt. will be able to lift pots & pans up to 20 lbs. p̄ 10 visits to allow Pt. to lift pots & pans & function indep. in her kitchen
2. Pt. will be able to reach items in an overhead cabinet up to 5 ft. 10 in. p̄ 10 Rx sessions to allow Pt. to reach items in her overhead kitchen cabinets at home & function indep. in her kitchen.

Writing Expected Outcomes Worksheet 2

Part I

1. A. Pt. (implied)
   B. will amb.
   C. c̄ straight cane
      on level surfaces
      on at least 5 stairs
   D. for 150 ft. ×2 (measurable)
      Indep. (observable)
      within 1 wk. (time span)
      so Pt.'s level of indep. at home ↑ (functional)
2. A. Pt.'s wife
   B. will transfer Pt. w/c↔supine in bed & w/c↔toilet
   C. w/c & bed must be present
   D. giving min. +1 assist to Pt. (observable)
      indep. (observable)
      p̄ 1 mo. of Rx & 5 sessions of family teaching (time span)
      so wife can care for Pt. at home (functional)
3. A. Pt.
   B. will transfer w/c↔floor
   C. it is assumed w/c is present
   D. Indep. (observable)
      within 3 mo. (time frame)
      so Pt. can safely play on the floor c̄ her siblings (functional)

Part II

1. Pt. will sit on the edge of a mat or chair s̄ falling for at least 10 min. p̄ 2 mo. of Rx to allow Pt. to more safely function at school.

2. Pt. will transfer supine↔sit, sit↔stand, & on/off toilet c̄ raised toilet seat indep. p̄ 2 wks. of Rx for Pt. to function indep. at home.
3. Pt. will propel w/c on level surfaces, including tiled & carpeted surfaces indep. p̄ 1 mo. of Rx to ↑ Pt.'s indep. at home.

Part III

1. Pt. will amb. c̄ a walker FWB as tolerated on level surfaces & 3 stairs c̄ a handrail in 2 wks. to allow Pt. to be safe in amb. as he returns home.
2. Pt. will transfer bed↔chair, sit↔stand & on/off commode indep. p̄ 2 wks. of Rx to allow Pt. to function at home alone.

Chapter 15

Writing Anticipated Goals: Worksheet 1

Part I

1. A. Pt. (implied)
   B. will ↑ Ⓡ shoulder flexion AROM
   C. (assumed you will measure AROM with a goniometer)
   D. to 0–90° (measurable)
      within 6 Rx sessions (time frame)
      to work toward Pt. reaching her overhead kitchen cupboards (functional)
2. A. Pt.
   B. will grasp object
   C. object will be in midline
   D. 3 out of 4 times (measurable)
      within 3 mo. (time span)
      to ↑ Pt.'s functional use of UEs during ADLs (functional)
3. A. Pt.
   B. will demonstrate good body mechanics
   C. by performance of tasks in obstacle course
   D. correct performance of at least 90% of tasks (measurable & observable)
      p̄ 3 Rx sessions (time span)
      to prevent further Pt. injury at work (functional)

Part II

1. Pt. will amb. c̄ a walker NWB Ⓛ LE ~100 ft. ×2 indep. on level surfaces only p̄ 1 wk. of Rx.
2. Pt.'s wife & son will transfer Pt. w/c↔supine in bed indep. p̄ 4 family training sessions within 2 wks. to care for Pt. at home.
3. Pt. will wrap residual limb c̄ 3 in. elastic wrap c̄ verbal cues for placement of elastic wrap p̄ 5 Rx sessions to prepare for prosthetic training.

Part III

1. (Case 1) Pt. will don & doff prosthesis c̄ contact guard of 1 person p̄ 1 wk. of Rx to assist c̄ sit↔stand transfers.

2. (Case 2) Pt. will be able to amb. c̄ straight cane c̄ at least 50% of body wt. shifted onto Ⓛ LE c̄ min. assist. of 1 & verbal cues p̄ 1 wk. of Rx.

3. (Case 3) Pt. will be pain free in prone on elbows position for 5 min. p̄ 2 Rx to progress Pt. toward indep. performance of ADLs.

Part IV

1. Degree (time span, measurable factors)

2. Degree (time span, measurable or observable factor; could be assumed to be 100% of the time correctly, some functional aspect of the goal is needed)

3. Audience, behavior (who will do what?), degree: functional aspect to the goal

Writing Anticipated Goals: Worksheet 2

Part I

1. A. Pt.
   B. will ↑ exercise tolerance
   C. p̄ amb. s̄ device for 150 ft.
   D. as demonstrated by max. ↑ of resp. rate of 5 breaths/min. (measurable)
   p̄ 6 Rx sessions (time span)
   to ↑ Pt. function in ADLS and IADLS at home (functional)

2. A. Pt.
   B. will be able to long sit
   C. propped c̄ a pillow or wedge
   D. maintaining good head position 0–45° of neck flexion
   (measurable/observable)
   for 1 min. (measurable)
   within 6 wks. of Rx (time span)
   to assist. c̄ Pt. function in the classroom (function)

3. A. Pt.
   B. will transfer supine↔sit on a mat
   C. mat must be there
   using rotation & pushing c̄ his UEs
   D. 1 out of 3 attempts correct (observable & measurable)
   within 1 mo. of Rx (time span)

Part II

1. Pt. will hold his head in midline while prone for 15 sec. within 3 mo. of Rx to assist Pt's ability to learn.

2. Pt. will roll supine↔prone on a mat indep. in 6–8 wks to assist. c̄ Pt's indep. at home.

3. Pt. will amb. 50% PWB Ⓡ LE on 5 stairs c̄ a walker c̄ min. assist. from his wife p̄ 1 wk. of Rx to ↑ Pt. function at home.

Part III

1. (Case 1)
   1. Pt. will be able to retrieve items 0.5 lbs. in wt. from the lower shelf of overhead cabinet p̄ 1 wk. of Rx.

2. Pt. will perform 7 reps of both UE PNF patterns within available AROM p̄ 1 wk. of Rx to progress Pt. to reaching into her cupboards.

3. ↑ Ⓡ shoulder flexion AROM to 100° p̄ 1 wk. of Rx to progress Pt. to reaching into her cupboards.

4. ↑ Ⓛ shoulder flexion AROM to 90° p̄ 1 wk. of Rx to progress Pt. to reaching into her cupboards.

5. ↑ strength throughout bilat. UEs to 3+/5 within available AROM p̄ 1 wk. of Rx to progress Pt. to reaching into her cupboards.

2. (Case 2) ↑ cervical rotation to 10° bilat. in 2 days to progress Pt. toward functional neck movement during ADLs.

3. (Case 3) Pt. will amb. NWB Ⓡ LE for 40 ft. ×2 on level surfaces c̄ min. assist. of 1 person in 1 wk.

Part IV

1. Degree (time span), Audience (could be assumed)

2. Degree (how much AROM is expected? Also, inclusion of function is needed), Audience (could be assumed)

3. Audience, Behavior (ambulate?), Condition (wt. bearing status?), Degree (time span, # of stairs)

Chapter 16

Writing the Intervention Plan: Worksheet 1

Part I

1. IP (intervention plan)

2. AG (anticipated goal)

3. IP

4. IP

5. AG

6. IP

7. AG

8. IP

9. AG

10. EO (expected outcome)

Part II

1. Pt. will be seen OD for hot pack for 20 min. to lumbar area to relax musculature prior to exercise.

2. Pt. will be seen 3×/wk. for continuous US at 1.0 W/cm² for 7 min. to Ⓡ upper trapezius

3. Pt. will be seen BID at B/S to progress Pt. through knee flex. & ext. strengthening exercise program for bilat. LEs (attached).

Part III

1. How often?
   For how long?
   Setting of the pump
   To what? (UE? LE? Right? Left?)
   For what purpose?

2. For how long?
   Which whirlpool?
   Temperature?
   Whirlpool additive used?
   To which part of the body?
   Some facilities list type of agitation (full, mild, direct, or indirect)?
   For what purpose?

Writing the Intervention Plan: Worksheet 2
Part I
1. IP (Intervention Plan)
2. EO (Expected Outcome)
3. IP
4. EO
5. IP
6. AG (Anticipated Goal)
7. AG (Pt.'s Expected Outcome is community ambulation)
8. AG
9. AG
10. IP
11. AG

Part II
1. 3×/wk as an OP: Pulsed US to Ⓡ shoulder at 1.5 W/cm² for 7 min. Mobilization to Ⓡ shoulder. Ice pack for 20 min. at end of Rx session. Pt. will be instructed in & given a copy of home exercise program for AROM to Ⓡ shoulder to ↑ Ⓡ shoulder function (attached). Will seek OT referral for ADL evaluation to assess Pt. function at home.
2. BID at B/S: Gait training c̄ axillary crutches NWB Ⓡ LE to prepare Pt. for indep at home. Transfer training sit↔stand, supine↔sit & on/off toilet to prepare Pt. for indep. at home. Resistive ROM exercise to LEs beginning c̄ 10 reps ea. exercise & ↑ to 30 reps ×3 sets to prepare Pt. for future amb. Pt. will be instructed in proper care of residual limb. Pt. will be instructed in wrapping his residual limb to prepare residual limb for future amb. training c̄ a prosthesis.

Final Review Worksheet Answers

Patient/Client Management Note: History, Systems Review, Tests and Measures, Evaluation, Diagnosis, Prognosis, Plan of Care SOAP Note: Problem, S, O, A, & P
Part I
11/08/2008: HISTORY: <u>Demographics</u>: Pt. is a 16 y.o. ♀ Pt. of Dr. Gungo. Medical dx: fx Ⓡ distal tibia & fx Ⓡ prox. humerus. ORIF Ⓡ proximal humerus on [date]. Cast applied to Ⓡ leg & sling applied Ⓡ UE. Pt. is Ⓡ-hand dominant. <u>Current Condition</u>: c/o pain Ⓡ ankle of an intensity of 10/10 when Ⓡ LE was initially in a dependent position (0 = no pain, 10 = worst possible pain). Pain Ⓡ ankle subsided p̄ Pt. put Ⓡ LE in a dependent position multiple times. Also c/o pain of 7/10 in Ⓡ shoulder c̄ Ⓡ elbow AAROM. Pt. reports difficulty feeding herself & cannot dress herself; states has not seen OT. Pt. was in a car accident c̄ 1 friend; the friend was driving & is currently in the community s̄ injury at this time. <u>Pt. Goals</u>: Pt. wants to return to school ASAP p̄ D/C. <u>Prior Level of Function</u>: Pt. was indep. in amb. & all ADLS prior to the accident. Has not used a w/c before. <u>Social hx</u>: Lives c̄ both parents. Parents both work so Pt. will be at home alone at D/C until she can go to school. Parents state insurance will rent a w/c for Pt. use until she is healed. <u>Employment status</u>: Pt. is a high school student. School is very academically challenging & competitive & Pt. does not believe she can stay out of school until she is healed. School is on 1 level c̄ no steps to enter. Distances between classrooms is 1500 ft. or less. Has 7 class periods/day. Floor surfaces are linoleum throughout the school. <u>Living environment</u>: Lives in a 1-story house c̄ 1 step at entrance s̄ handrail. Home has carpeted floor surfaces throughout. General health status: Pt. & parents report Pt. on swim team at school; swims daily all year & general health is good. <u>Social/health habits</u>: Pt. does not smoke or drink ETOH. Family health hx: Htn. both parents controlled by medication. <u>Pt.'s medical/surgical hx</u>: No previous hospitalizations or serious illnesses. <u>Medications</u>: Pt. is currently taking [pain medication]; takes no other medications regularly. Other clinical tests: X-ray: good alignment of Ⓡ LE fx in cast & of Ⓡ humerus p̄ surgery.

SYSTEMS REVIEW: <u>Cardiopulmonary</u>: not impaired. BP 110/70. HR 70 bpm. Resp. rate 12 breaths/min. No edema noted. <u>Integumentary</u>: impaired. Disruption of skin at incision site Ⓡ upper arm. Continuity of skin color: bruising noted Ⓡ UE & Ⓡ foot. Pliability: not impaired Ⓛ extremities; Ⓡ extremities not tested this date. <u>Musculoskeletal</u>: impaired. Gross symmetry not impaired sitting; cannot stand. Gross ROM impaired Ⓡ UE & LE. Gross strength impaired Ⓡ UE & LE. Height: 5' 6", weight 125 lbs. <u>Neuromuscular</u>: Gait impaired. Locomotion impaired. Balance not impaired sitting; cannot stand. Motor function not impaired. <u>Communication</u>: not impaired; age-appropriate. <u>Cognition</u>: not impaired; oriented ×3. <u>Learning barriers</u>: none. <u>Learning style</u>: Pt. best learns by listening as she tries an activity. <u>Education needs</u>: healing process of incision, adaptation of home to w/c, w/c management, w/c propulsion, ADLs, safety c̄ w/c; home exercise program for Ⓡ UE. ─────────

TESTS & MEASURES: <u>Transfers</u>: sit↔stand & w/c↔bed c̄ max. assist of 1 NWB Ⓡ LE & UE. Supine ↔sit c̄ mod. assist of 1 person. Toilet transfers not tested this date due to Pt. fatigue. <u>W/c Management</u>: Unable to manage Ⓡ w/c brakes or leg rest. <u>W/c propulsion</u>:

propelled w/c 10 ft. using Ⓛ LE & UE c̄ min. assist. of 1 person & verbal cues. Was too exhausted to continue further. Ⓛ LE & UE: WNL AROM & strength throughout. Ⓡ UE: Bruising noted throughout entire Ⓡ UE. Ⓡ shoulder not examined further due to recent fx. Ⓡ elbow AAROM: 30–70°. Ⓡ hand & wrist AROM WNL when Pt. is given verbal cues to complete full ROM; performed very slowly. Strength Ⓡ biceps and triceps: 2/5. Strength of musculature controlling Ⓡ wrist & hand is 3/5. Ⓡ LE: Bruising noted Ⓡ toes. Toes warm & color WNL. AROM WNL at hip & knee. Strength 5/5 Ⓡ hip & knee musculature. Able to wiggle toes. Short leg cast Ⓡ ankle & foot so not further examined this date. Trunk: Bruising noted Ⓡ posterior trunk. ———————

EVALUATION: Rigorous AROM Ⓡ elbow, wrist, & hand are needed to prevent loss of strength & ROM. Pt.'s lack of mobility is due to inability to use Ⓡ extremities due to recent fx. A referral to OT is essential to Pt.'s rehab. process to assist. her c̄ eating, bathing, dressing, & managing items for return to school in a w/c. ———————
DIAGNOSIS: Practice Pattern Musculoskeletal G: Impaired Joint Mobility, Muscle Performance & ROM Associated c̄ Fx. ———————
PROGNOSIS: Pt. has excellent rehab. potential. Will be able to return home & to school c̄ 2 wks. of rehab. Pt. cannot stay at home alone until she becomes indep. in w/c propulsion & transfers. Pt. will need assist. in propelling her w/c distances over 500 ft. at school. ———————

EXPECTED OUTCOMES: to be achieved p̄ 2 wks. of PT ———————
1. Pt. will indep. transfer supine↔sit, sit↔stand, w/c↔bed, on/off toilet NWB Ⓡ LE & UE to be functional at home & school.
2. Pt. will indep. manage w/c brakes & footrests to function at home & school.
3. Pt. will propel w/c for 500 ft. ×2 indep. using Ⓛ UE & LE to function at school.
4. Pt. will prevent loss of function in Ⓡ elbow, wrist, & fingers to maximize UE function p̄ Ⓡ humerus is healed.

ANTICIPATED GOALS: To be achieved p̄ 1 wk. of PT
1. Pt. will transfer supine↔sit c̄ verbal cues.
2. Pt. will transfer sit↔stand c̄ min. assist. of 1.
3. Pt. will transfer w/c↔bed & on/off toilet c̄ mod. assist. of 1 person.
4. Pt. will manage w/c brakes & footrest using an extended Ⓡ brake lever c̄ verbal cues.
5. Pt. will propel w/c for ~100 ft. using Ⓛ UE & LE.
6. Pt. will be indep. in performing home exercise program for AROM of Ⓡ elbow, wrist & fingers to allow for function of Ⓡ UE p̄ Ⓡ humerus is healed.

INTERVENTION PLAN: Will see Pt. BID at B/S. Will instruct Pt. in transfers supine↔sit, sit↔stand, w/c↔bed & on/off toilet. Will instruct Pt. in w/c management & propulsion so Pt. can become independent in her home & school settings. Will teach Pt. a home

exercise program for AROM to Ⓡ elbow, wrist, & fingers & will give Pt. a copy of program (attached). Once indep., Pt. will perform the exercise program TID, OD c̄ PT supervision to encourage ↑ in AROM Ⓡ elbow, wrist & fingers & BID indep. ——————— [your name], SPT/

Part II
PROBLEM: Pt. is a 16 y.o. ♀ Pt. of Dr. Gungo. Pt. is Ⓡ-hand dominant. Medical dx: fx Ⓡ distal tibia & fx Ⓡ prox. humerus. ORIF Ⓡ proximal humerus on [date]. Cast applied to Ⓡ leg & sling applied Ⓡ UE. Other clinical tests: X-ray: good alignment of Ⓡ LE fx in cast & of Ⓡ humerus p̄ surgery. Medications: Pt. is currently taking [pain medication]; takes no other medications regularly. ———————

S: Current Condition: c/o pain Ⓡ ankle of an intensity of 10/10 when Ⓡ LE was initially in a dependent position (0 = no pain, 10 = worst possible pain). Pain Ⓡ ankle subsided p̄ Pt. put Ⓡ LE in a dependent position multiple times. Also c/o pain of 7/10 in Ⓡ shoulder c̄ Ⓡ elbow AAROM. Pt. reports difficulty feeding herself & cannot dress herself; states has not seen OT. Pt. was in a car accident c̄ 1 friend; the friend was driving & is currently in the community s̄ injury at this time. Prior level of function: Pt. was indep. in amb. & all ADLs prior to accident. Never used a w/c PTA. Pt. goals: Pt. wants to return to school ASAP p̄ D/C. Social hx: Lives c̄ both parents. Parents both work so Pt. will be at home alone at D/C until she can go to school. Parents state insurance will rent a w/c for Pt. use until she is healed. Employment status: Pt. is a high school student. School is very academically challenging & competitive & Pt. does not believe she can stay out of school until she is healed. School is on 1 level c̄ no steps to enter. Distances between classrooms 1500 ft. or less. Has 7 class periods/day. Floor surfaces are linoleum throughout the school. Living environment: Lives in a 1-story house c̄ 1 step at entrance s̄ handrail. Home has carpeted floor surfaces throughout. General health status: Pt. & parents report Pt. on swim team at school; swims daily all year & general health is good. Social/health habits: Pt. does not smoke or drink ETOH. Family health hx: Htn. both parents controlled by medication. Pt.'s medical/surgical hx: No previous hospitalizations or serious illnesses. ———————

O: SYSTEMS REVIEW: Cardiopulmonary: not impaired. BP 110/70. HR 70 bpm. Resp. rate 12/breaths min. No edema noted. Integumentary: impaired. Disruption of skin at incision site Ⓡ upper arm. Continuity of skin color: bruising noted Ⓡ UE & Ⓡ foot. Pliability: not impaired Ⓛ extremities; Ⓡ extremities not tested this date. Musculoskeletal: impaired. Gross symmetry not impaired sitting; cannot stand. Gross ROM: impaired Ⓡ UE & LE. Gross strength: impaired Ⓡ UE & LE. Height 5′ 6″, weight 125 lbs. Neuromuscular: Gait impaired. Locomotion impaired. Balance not impaired sitting; cannot stand. Motor function not impaired. <u>Communication</u>: not impaired; age-appropriate. <u>Cognition</u>: not impaired; oriented ×3. <u>Learning barriers</u>: none. <u>Learning style</u>: Pt. best learns by listening as she tries an activity. <u>Education needs</u>: healing process of incision, adaptation of home to w/c, w/c management, w/c propulsion, ADLs, safety c̄ w/c, home exercise program for Ⓡ UE.

TESTS & MEASURES: <u>Transfers</u>: sit↔stand & w/c↔bed c̄ max. assist of 1 NWB Ⓡ LE & UE. Supine↔sit c̄ mod. assist. of 1 person. Toilet transfers not tested this date due to Pt. fatigue. <u>W/c Management</u>: Unable to manage Ⓡ w/c brakes or leg rest. <u>W/c propulsion</u>: propelled w/c 10 ft. using Ⓛ LE & UE c̄ min. assist. of 1 person & verbal cues. Was too exhausted to continue further. Ⓛ LE & UE: WNL AROM & strength throughout. Ⓡ UE: Bruising noted throughout entire Ⓡ UE. Ⓡ shoulder not examined further due to recent fx. Ⓡ elbow AAROM: 30–70°. Ⓡ hand & wrist AROM WNL when Pt. is given verbal cues to complete full ROM; performed very slowly. Strength Ⓡ biceps & triceps: 2/5. Strength of musculature controlling Ⓡ wrist & hand is 3/5. Ⓡ LE: Bruising noted Ⓡ toes. Toes warm & color WNL. AROM WNL at hip & knee. Strength 5/5 Ⓡ hip & knee musculature. Able to wiggle toes. Short leg cast Ⓡ ankle & foot so not further examined this date. Trunk: Bruising noted Ⓡ posterior trunk. ———

A: EVALUATION: Rigorous AROM Ⓡ elbow, wrist, & hand are needed to prevent loss of strength & ROM. Pt.'s lack of mobility is due to inability to use Ⓡ extremities due to recent fx. A referral to OT is essential to Pt.'s rehab. process to assist. her c̄ eating, bathing, dressing, & managing items for return to school in a w/c. DIAGNOSIS: Practice Pattern Musculoskeletal G: Impaired Joint Mobility, Muscle Performance & ROM Associated c̄ Fx. PROGNOSIS: Pt. has excellent rehab. potential. Will be able to return home & to school c̄ 2 wks. of rehab. Pt. cannot stay at home alone until she becomes indep. in w/c propulsion & transfers. Pt. will need assist. in propelling her w/c distances over 500 ft. at school. ———

P: EXPECTED OUTCOMES: to be achieved p̄ 2 wks. of PT———

1. Pt. will indep. transfer supine↔sit, sit↔stand, w/c↔bed, on/off toilet NWB Ⓡ LE & UE to be functional at home & school.
2. Pt. will indep. manage w/c brakes & footrests to function at home & school.
3. Pt. will propel w/c for 500 ft. ×2 indep. using Ⓛ UE & LE to function at school.
4. Pt. will prevent loss of function in Ⓡ elbow, wrist, & fingers to maximize UE function p̄ Ⓡ humerus is healed.

ANTICIPATED GOALS: To be achieved p̄ 1 wk. of PT
1. Pt. will transfer supine↔sit c̄ verbal cues.
2. Pt. will transfer sit↔stand c̄ min. assist. of 1.
3. Pt. will transfer w/c↔bed & on/off toilet c̄ mod. assist. of 1 person.

4. Pt. will manage w/c brakes & footrest using an extended Ⓡ brake lever c̄ verbal cues.
5. Pt. will propel w/c for ~100 ft. using Ⓛ UE & LE.
6. Pt. will be indep. in performing home exercise program for AROM of Ⓡ elbow, wrist & fingers to allow for function of Ⓡ UE p̄ Ⓡ humerus is healed.

INTERVENTION PLAN: Will see Pt. BID at B/S. Will instruct Pt. in transfers supine↔sit, sit↔stand, w/c↔bed & on/off toilet. Will instruct Pt. in w/c management & propulsion so Pt. can become independent in her home & school settings. Will teach Pt. a home exercise program for AROM to Ⓡ elbow, wrist, & fingers & will give Pt. a copy of program (attached). Once indep., Pt. will perform the exercise program TID, OD c̄ PT supervision to encourage ↑ in AROM Ⓡ elbow, wrist & fingers & BID indep. ——————————
[your name], SPT/

Chapter 22

1a. **activities and participation.** *Combing her hair* and *washing her windows* are part of the domain of activities and participation because they are tasks or actions executed by an individual and/or involvement in a life situation.

1b. **d.** This is the letter in the ICF coding system that represents items in the domain of activities and participation.

2. **activity limitation/participation restriction.** Sophia's *inability to work for the last few months at her job as a factory worker* is an activity limitation/participation restriction because it represents some level of difficulty in performing a task or action, or to participate in a life situation. Using ICF's broad definition, this can also be understood as a disability.

3a. **body function.** *Loss of power of the abductors and lateral rotators of the glenohumeral joint* would fall under the domain of body function because it describes the physiology of an organ system or body part. This case describes physiologic function of muscles, which are part of the musculoskeletal system.

3b. **b.** This is the letter in the ICF coding system that represents items in the domain of body function.

4a. **body structure.** The *partial tear of the supraspinatus tendon* would fall under the domain of Body Structure because this is a description that refers to the anatomical status of a body part.

4b. **s.** This is the letter in the ICF coding system that represents items in the domain of body structure.

5. **impairments.** *Deficits in passive mobility of glenohumeral flexion, loss of power in all the abductor and lateral rotator muscles of the shoulder, "stabbing" shoulder pain* and *a partial tear of the supraspinatus* *tendon* all describe deficits in either body structure (i.e., partial tear of the supraspinatus tendon) or body function (i.e., deficits in mobility of the shoulder, loss of muscle power, and shoulder pain). Deficits in the domains of body structure or body function are known as impairments if they differ from generally accepted norms found in persons without health conditions. Using ICF's broad definition, these can also be understood as disabilities.

6a. environmental factor. *Her employer refuses to let her return to work because he feels she is exaggerating the amount of shoulder pain she experiences.* This phrase would be categorized under the environmental factor domain because it describes attitude of an authority figure in Sophia's environment. In addition to societal expectations and attitudes, environmental factors include the physical environment of the person.

6b. e. This is the letter in the ICF coding system that represents items in the domain of environmental factors.

7. environmental barrier. *Her work station is currently too high for her to reach without shoulder pain.* This phrase describes an environmental barrier because it is something in her physical environment that impedes her health status.

8. environmental facilitator. *Reconfiguring her work station by lowering it* would be a change in the physical environment that would promote an improvement of her health status and is therefore an environmental facilitator.

9. performance qualifier. *Reaching objects on the shelves of her kitchen cabinets* is a description of how an activity/participation occurs in Sophia's daily life situation in her typical environment (i.e., her own kitchen). Therefore, coding this description requires the use of a performance qualifier.

10. capacity qualifier. *Reaching objects on the shelves of your clinic* is a description of how an activity/participation occurs in an idealized environment (i.e., your clinic). The clinic is a standardized environment where environmental barriers have been minimized so that Sophia can perform the activity at her highest probable level. Therefore, coding this description requires the use of a capacity qualifier.

11. disability. *Loss of power in all of the abductor and lateral rotator muscles of the glenohumeral joint, a partial tear of the supraspinatus tendon, difficulty combing her hair* and *washing her windows* are examples of impairments (i.e., loss of muscle power and a partial tear of her supraspinatus tendon) and activity limitations/participation restrictions (i.e., difficulty combing her hair and washing windows). This mix of impairments and activity limitations/participation restrictions would all be considered disabilities in the broad definition used by ICF.

12. health conditions. The *impingement syndrome of her rotator cuff*, and *inflammation in her supraspinatus tendon* are both examples of health conditions. They are typically considered diseases or medical disorders.

B | Summary of the Patient/ Client Management Note Contents

Initial Note

History

- **Demographics**/Identifying information (patient's name, address, admission date, date of birth, sex, dominant hand, race, ethnicity, language, education level, advance directive preferences, referral source, and reasons for referral to therapy).
- **Current conditions/chief complaints** (onset date of the problem, any incident that caused or contributed to the onset of the problem, prior history of similar problems, how the patient is caring for the problem, what makes the problem better and worse, patient goals for therapy, and any other practitioner the patient is seeing for the problem).
- **Patient goals:** This includes the patient/client and sometimes family goals for therapy as told to the therapist by the patient/client or family/caretaker in cases where the patient cannot speak for him/herself.
- **Prior level of function:** This describes the patient's level of function prior to the most recent onset of his/her current condition or complaints. If the patient has a chronic condition, this includes the level of function prior to the most recent onset or exacerbation of his/her symptoms.
- **Social history** (cultural/religious beliefs that might affect care, the person(s) with whom the patient lived prior to admission and will live with at discharge, available social and physical supports the patient has now and will have at discharge, and the availability of a caregiver).
- **Employment status** (full time or part time, inside or outside of the home, retired or a student, description of the workplace and/or workplace demands)
- **Living environment** (devices and equipment the patient uses, the type of residence, information about the environment such as stairs or ramps available, and past use of community services such as day services or program, home-health services, homemaking services, hospice, Meals on Wheels, mental health services, respiratory therapy, or one of the rehabilitation therapies)
- **General health status** (patient's rating of his or her health and whether the patient has experienced any major life changes during the past year)
- **Social/health habits** (past and current alcohol and tobacco use and exercise habits)

- **Family health history** (family history of heart disease, hypertension, stroke, diabetes, cancer, psychological conditions, arthritis, osteoporosis, and other conditions)
- **Patient's medical/surgical history**
- **Functional status/activity level** (everything from bed mobility, transfers, gait, self-care, home management, and community and work activities that apply to the patient's current situation or condition)
- **Medications** the patient takes
- **Growth and development** (developmental history of a patient, if applicable)
- **Other clinical tests** (laboratory or radiologic tests, the dates of those tests, and the findings of those tests)

Systems Review

- **Cardiovascular/Pulmonary** (heart rate, respiratory rate, blood pressure, or edema): listed as impaired or not impaired; individual measurements of heart rate, blood pressure, respiratory rate, and a general description of edema are listed.
- **Integumentary System** (integumentary disruption, continuity of skin color, skin pliability or texture): listed as impaired or not impaired.
- **Musculoskeletal System:** gross symmetry during standing, sitting, and activities; gross range of motion; gross muscle strength; each listed as impaired or unimpaired; height and weight are recorded.
- **Neuromuscular System:** gait, locomotion (transfers, bed mobility), balance, and motor function (motor control, motor learning) are each listed as impaired or unimpaired.
- **Communication Style or Abilities** (including age-appropriate communication): listed as impaired or unimpaired.
- **Affect** (emotional/behavioral responses): listed as impaired or unimpaired.
- **Cognition** (whether the patient is oriented to person, place, and time [oriented ×3] or the patient's level of consciousness): listed as impaired or unimpaired.
- **Learning Barriers:** notes difficulty with vision or hearing, inability to read, inability to understand what is read, language barriers (needs an interpreter), and any other learning barrier noted by the therapist.
- **Learning Style:** notes how the patient/client best learns (pictures, reading, listening, demonstration, other).

- **Education Needs:** reports areas in which the patient needs more education or information (disease process, safety, use of devices/equipment, activities of daily living, exercise program, recovery and healing process, and other education needs).

Tests and Measures

Items in the Tests and Measures section should have the following attributes:

- Items should be a result of tests and measures performed by the therapist or an observation made by the therapist.
- Items should be listed in a subcategory that organizes the information in a logical manner, either by test performed or functional activity observed, or by part of the body reported.

Evaluation

The Evaluation subsection may include any of the following:

- The **relatioship among impairments, functional deficits, and disability.** This can include a description of how impairments relate to the functional deficits and/or a description of how functional deficits keep the patient from functioning in his specific environment.
- **Justifications of decisions made by the therapist** in terms of Expected Outcomes, Anticipated Goals set, or the interventions included in the Intervention Plan and the relationship among these parts of the Plan of Care.
- **Inconsistencies** between examination findings.
- **Further testing needed.**
- **Referral to another practitioner.**
- A **justification of unusual expected outcomes or anticipated goals.**
- A **discussion of the patient's progress in therapy** (why the patient failed to progress as quickly as predicted, why a patient suddenly regressed, or why a patient suddenly progressed more quickly than predicted).
- A **justification for further therapy** for a patient who appears relatively independent with one functional activity.
- A discussion or listing of **future services needed.**

Diagnosis

The Diagnosis section may include any of the following:

- Placement of patient's deficits **in primary and at times secondary practice patterns/movement dysfunction diagnostic categories**
- A brief **summary of the examination findings that led the therapist to place the patient in a specific practice pattern or movement dysfunction diagnosis**

Prognosis

The Prognosis section may include any of the following:

- The patient's **rehabilitation potential**
- A **prediction of a level of improvement** in function and the **amount of time needed** to reach that level
- A discussion of **factors influencing the prognosis,** such as living environment, patient's condition prior to the onset of the current therapy diagnosis, and current illnesses or medical conditions

Expected Outcomes

1. Outcomes state the long-term expected outcomes of therapy.
2. Outcomes are generally functional.
3. Outcomes are based on discussion during the Diagnosis and Prognosis parts of the note.
4. Outcomes are the basis for setting Anticipated Goals.

Components of Expected Outcomes

1. **Audience:** The patient, a family member, or the patient with a family member (sometimes implied).
2. **Behavior:** An action verb, often followed by the object of the behavior.
3. **Condition:** The circumstances under which the behavior must be done or the conditions necessary for the behavior to occur (sometimes implied).
4. **Degree:** The minimal number, the percentage or proportion, limitation or departure from a fixed standard, or distinguishing features of successful performance; always includes a time span for achievement of the outcome and a tie to the patient's function in his environment.

Anticipated Goals

1. Goals are the steps along the way to achieving Expected Outcomes.
2. Goals are based on the Expected Outcomes.
3. Goals serve as the basis for setting the Intervention Plan.

The components of Anticipated Goals are the same as those of Expected Outcomes. Anticipated Goals differ from Expected Outcomes in the following ways:

1. The time span is not as long.
2. Anticipated goals are not as frequently expressed in functional terms in some facilities.
3. Anticipated goals are frequently revised.

Intervention Plan

The Intervention Plan must include the following information:

1. Frequency per day or per week that the patient will be seen (or the total number of visits that the therapist will see the patient)

2. The intervention the patient will receive

Also frequently included are the following:

1. The location of the intervention
2. The intervention progression
3. Plans for further examination or re-examination
4. Plans for discharge
5. Plans for patient and/or family education
6. Equipment needs and equipment ordered for or sold to the patient
7. Interventions received during the first visit/day of therapy and the patient's reaction to these interventions.

Progress Note

History
Includes updates or additional information regarding the patient's status since the most recent note was written.

Systems Review
Usually not included unless the patient's condition changes.

Tests and Measures
Tests and measures are updated or added to the information reported in the initial note or last progress note.

Evaluation
This is part of a progress note if referral to another practitioner has been made or recommended, or if the patient's condition or examination findings indicate that the patient has different problems than stated in the initial note or past progress notes.

Diagnosis
Diagnosis is usually discussed in a progress note only if the therapy diagnosis has changed or if the patient's functional activities or impairments change to fit a different primary or secondary practice pattern or movement dysfunction category.

Prognosis
The prognosis is usually mentioned only if the prognosis changes as a result of a change in the patient's condition.

Expected Outcomes
Expected Outcomes usually are not addressed in progress notes unless they have been achieved or need to be revised.

Anticipated Goals
Progress notes refer to the Anticipated Goals achieved and set new Anticipated Goals. If a goal has not yet been achieved, the notes comment on the reason the Anticipated Goal has not been achieved and reset the goal to

make it more reasonable or restate the same goal to include a new time span.

Intervention Plan
The Intervention Plan needs to be revised as the patient's condition is re-examined and new Anticipated Goals are set. Interventions received during the visit in which the re-examination and re-evaluation were completed, and the patient's reaction to these interventions, should be listed.

Discharge Notes

History
The History includes updates or additional information regarding the patient's status since the most recent note was written *or* completely summarizes the history of the patient from the initial note through discharge, whether the patient feels the goals set were achieved, and whether the patient feels ready to function at home or work.

Systems Review
In a discharge note, the Systems Review is either not mentioned at all *or* the note completely summarizes the Systems Review written in the initial note.

Tests and Measures
The discharge note updates the patient's status since the last note was written *or* completely summarizes the patient's condition upon discharge from the facility (more similar to the initial note in format and length).

Evaluation
The evaluation may include the following:

1. A discussion of any remaining functional limitations
2. A discussion of suggested further therapy
3. A discussion of whether or not the patient achieved the Expected Outcomes and Anticipated Goals
4. Referrals made to other health professionals

Diagnosis
The diagnosis may include a discussion of the progression of the patient through diagnostic categories or movement dysfunction diagnoses, *or* a diagnosis section similar to the initial note.

Prognosis
The prognosis may include a prognosis for meeting an Expected Outcome when the patient completes all therapy for this episode of care.

Expected Outcomes
The discharge summary indicates which of the Expected Outcomes have been achieved and which have not (and why not).

Anticipated Goals

In some facilities, comments are made on the most recently set Anticipated Goals and why they were or were not achieved. In other facilities, no comment is made on the Anticipated Goals.

Intervention Plan

The following information should be briefly stated:

1. Interventions delivered
2. If instruction in a home program was done and the patient's/caregiver's level of independence in the program
3. If any other type of instruction of the patient or family was performed and the level of learning that occurred (in observable terms)

4. If the patient was sold any type of equipment
5. If written instructions for any equipment sold to the patient were given
6. The number of times the patient was seen in therapy
7. Any instances of the patient skipping or canceling treatment sessions
8. If and when the patient was not seen or was put on hold, and why
9. To where the patient was discharged
10. The reason for discharge from PT
11. Recommendations for follow-up interventions or care given to the patient

Bibliography

1. American Physical Therapy Association: Guide to Physical Therapist Practice, ed. 2, and CD-ROM. American Physical Therapy Association, Alexandria, VA, 2003.
2. Defensible Documentation for Patient/Client Management. Accessed at http://www.apta.org/AM/Template.cfm?Section=Documentation4&Template=/MembersOnly.cfm&ContentID=37776 on March 9, 2007.
3. American Physical Therapy Association: Guidelines: Physical Therapy Documentation of Patient/Client Management. Accessed at http://www.apta.org/AM/Template.cfm?Section=Home&TEMPLATE=/CM/ ContentDisplay.cfm& CONTENTID=31688 on March 9, 2007.

C Summary of the SOAP Note Contents*

Initial Note

Problem

The Problem part of the note contains the following:

- **Medical diagnosis/present conditions/diseases** affecting the present condition/treatment
- **Demographic information** (patient's name, address, admission date, date of birth, sex, dominant hand, race, ethnicity, language, education level, advance directive preferences, referral source, and reasons for referral to therapy)
- **Recent or past surgeries** affecting the present condition/treatment
- **Past conditions/diseases** affecting the present condition/treatment
- **Medical test results** affecting the present condition/treatment
- **Medication list** if you obtained this list from the patient's medical record and not from the patient

Subjective (S)

The Subjective part of the note contains information that the patient and/or significant others tell the therapist or assistant, such as:

- **Current conditions/chief complaints** (the onset date of the problem, any incident that caused or contributed to the onset of the problem, prior history of similar problems, how the patient is caring for the problem, what makes the problem better and worse, and any other practitioner the patient is seeing for the problem).
- **Prior level of function** of the patient prior to the most recent onset of his current condition or complaints. If the patient has a chronic condition, this includes the level of function prior to the most recent onset or exacerbation of his/her symptoms.
- **Patient goals** for therapy.
- **Social history** (cultural/religious beliefs that might affect care, the person(s) with whom the patient lived prior to admission and will live with at discharge, available social and physical supports the patient has now and will have at discharge, and the availability of a caregiver).
- **Employment status** (full time or part time, inside or outside of the home, retired or student, and work place demands and set-up).

- **Living environment** (devices and equipment the patient uses, the type of residence in which the patient lives, information about the living environment such as stairs or ramps available, past use of community services including day services or programs, home-health services, homemaking services, hospice, Meals on Wheels, mental health services, respiratory therapy, or one of the rehabilitation therapies).
- **General health status** (rating of the patient's health and whether the patient has experienced any major life changes during the past year).
- **Social/health habits** (past and current alcohol and tobacco use and exercise habits).
- **Family health history** (heart disease, hypertension, stroke, diabetes, cancer, psychological conditions, arthritis, osteoporosis, and other conditions).
- **Functional status/activity level** (activities that the patient can no longer perform as a result of the patient's current condition; includes bed mobility, transfers, gait, self-care, home management, and community and work activities that apply to the patient's current situation or condition).
- **Patient's medical/surgical history.**
- **Medications** that the patient currently takes, if this list is obtained from the patient.
- **Growth and development** (developmental history of a patient; most applicable to pediatric patients).
- **Other clinical tests** (laboratory or radiologic tests, the dates of those tests, and the findings of those tests, if these test results are obtained from the patient interview).
- **Response to treatment interventions.**

Objective (O)

The Objective part of the note must include the following:

Systems Review

- **Cardiovascular/Pulmonary** (heart rate, respiratory rate, blood pressure or edema): listed as impaired or not impaired; individual measurements of heart rate, blood pressure, respiratory rate, and a general description of edema are listed.
- **Integumentary System** (integumentary disruption, continuity of skin color, skin pliability or texture): listed as impaired or not impaired.

---

*The SOAP Note format is not recommended by the American Physical Therapy Association.

- **Musculoskeletal System:** gross symmetry during standing, sitting, and activities; gross range of motion; gross muscle strength. Each are listed as impaired or unimpaired; height and weight are recorded.
- **Neuromuscular System:** gait, locomotion (transfers, bed mobility), balance, and motor function (motor control, motor learning). Each are listed as impaired or unimpaired.
- **Communication Style or Abilities** (including age-appropriate communication): listed as impaired or unimpaired.
- **Affect** (emotional and behavioral responses): listed as impaired or unimpaired.
- **Cognition** (whether the patient is oriented to person, place and time [oriented ×3] or the patient's level of consciousness): listed as impaired or unimpaired.
- **Learning Barriers:** notes difficulty with vision or hearing, inability to read, inability to understand what is read, language barriers (needs an interpreter), and any other learning barrier noted by the therapist.
- **Learning Style:** notes how the patient/client best learns (pictures, reading, listening, demonstration, other).
- **Education Needs:** reports areas in which the patient needs more education or information (disease process, safety, use of devices/equipment, activities of daily living, exercise program, recovery/healing process, and other education needs).

Tests and Measures

The Objective part of the note also includes any of the following information (depending on the individual clinical facility):

1. Information that is a result of tests and measures (must be measurable and reproducible data; may use database, flow sheets, or charts, and summarize data under Objective).
2. Part of the interventions already given to a patient (particularly specific exercises taught to the patient, the level of independence in performing the exercises, number of repetitions tolerated, positions used, modifications necessary).
3. Functional information; this information is usually stated first in the Objective part of the note.

Items in the Objective section should meet the following criteria:

- Items should be a result of tests and measures performed by the therapist or an observation made by the therapist.
- Items should be listed in a subcategory that organizes the information in a logical manner, either by test performed/functional activity observed or by part of the body reported.

Assessment (A)

The Assessment part of the note has three subsections: Evaluation, Diagnosis, and Prognosis.

Evaluation

The Evaluation subsection may include any of the following:

- The **relationship among impairments, functional deficits, and disability.** This can include a description of how impairments relate to the functional deficits and/or a description of how functional deficits keep the patient from functioning in his or her specific environment.
- **Justifications of decisions made by the therapist** in terms of Expected Outcomes, Anticipated Goals set or the interventions included in the Intervention Plan and the relationship among these parts of the Plan of Care.
- **Inconsistencies** between examination findings.
- **Further testing needed.**
- **Referral to another practitioner.**
- A **justification of unusual Expected Outcomes or Anticipated Goals.**
- A **discussion of the patient's progress in therapy** (why the patient failed to progress as quickly as predicted, why the patient suddenly regressed, or why the patient suddenly progressed more quickly than predicted).
- A **justification for further therapy** for a patient who appears relatively independent with one functional activity.
- A discussion or listing of **future services needed.**

Diagnosis

The Diagnosis subsection may include any of the following:

- Placement of patient's deficits **in primary and at times secondary practice patterns/movement dysfunction diagnostic categories**
- A brief **summary of the examination findings that led the therapist to place the patient in a specific practice pattern or movement dysfunction diagnosis**

Prognosis

The Prognosis subsection may include any of the following:

- The patient's **rehabilitation potential**
- A **prediction of a level of improvement** in function and the **amount of time needed** to reach that level
- A discussion of **factors influencing the prognosis,** such as living environment, patient's condition prior to the onset of the current therapy diagnosis, and current illnesses or medical conditions

Plan of Care (P)

The Plan of Care part of the note has three subsections: Expected Outcomes, Anticipated Goals, and Interventions or Intervention Plan.

Expected Outcomes

1. Outcomes state the long-term expected outcomes of therapy.
2. Outcomes are generally functional.

3. Outcomes are based on discussion during the Diagnosis and Prognosis parts of the note.
4. Outcomes are the basis for setting Anticipated Goals.

Components of Expected Outcomes
1. **Audience:** The patient, a family member, or the patient with a family member (sometimes implied)
2. **Behavior:** An action verb, often followed by the object of the behavior
3. **Condition:** The circumstances under which the behavior must be done or the conditions necessary for the behavior to occur (sometimes implied)
4. **Degree:** The minimal number, the percentage or proportion, limitation or departure from a fixed standard, or distinguishing features of successful performance; always includes a time span for achievement of the outcome and a tie to the patient's function in his environment

Anticipated Goals
1. Goals are the steps along the way to achieving Expected Outcomes.
2. Goals are based on the Expected Outcomes.
3. Goals serve as the basis for setting the Intervention Plan.

The components of Anticipated Goals are the same as those of Expected Outcomes. Anticipated Goals differ from Expected Outcomes in the following ways:

1. The time span is not as long.
2. Anticipated Goals are not as frequently expressed in functional terms in some facilities.
3. Anticipated Goals are frequently revised.

Intervention Plan
The Intervention Plan must include the following information:

1. Frequency per day or per week that the patient will be seen (or the total number of visits that the therapist will see the patient).
2. The intervention the patient will receive.

Also frequently included are the following:

1. The location of the intervention
2. The intervention progression
3. Plans for further examination or re-examination
4. Plans for discharge
5. Plans for patient and/or family education
6. Equipment needs and equipment ordered for or sold to the patient
7. Interventions received during the first visit/day of therapy and the patient's reaction to these interventions

Progress Notes

Problem
The Problem section is included in the note only if there are updates or additional information regarding the medical diagnosis, test results, or medications since the most recent note was written.

Subjective (S)
Progress notes include updates or additional information regarding the patient's status since the most recent note was written.

Objective (O)
Systems Review
System Review is usually not included unless the patient's condition changes.

Reporting of Tests and Measures
Tests and Measures are updated or added to the information reported in the initial note or last progress note.

Assessment (A)
Evaluation
This is part of a progress note if referral to another practitioner has been made or recommended, or if the patient's condition or examination findings indicate that the patient has different problems than stated in the initial note or past progress notes.

Diagnosis
Diagnosis is usually discussed in a progress note only if the therapy diagnosis has changed or if the patient's functional activities or impairments change to fit a different primary or secondary practice pattern or movement dysfunction category.

Prognosis
The prognosis is usually mentioned only if the prognosis changes as a result of a change in the patient's condition.

Plan of Care (P)
Expected Outcomes
Expected Outcomes usually are not addressed in progress notes unless they have been achieved or need to be revised.

Anticipated Goals
Progress notes refer to the Anticipated Goals achieved and set new Anticipated Goals. If a goal has not yet been achieved, the notes comment on the reason the Anticipated Goal has not been achieved and reset the goal to make it more reasonable, or restate the same goal to include a new time span.

Intervention Plan
The Intervention Plan needs to be revised as the patient's condition is re-examined and new Anticipated Goals are set. Interventions received during the the visit in which the re-examination and re-evaluation were completed

and the patient's reaction to these interventions should be listed.

Discharge Notes

Problem

The Problem section of the Discharge Notes includes updates or additional information regarding the patient's medical status, test results, or medications since the most recent note was written, *or* completely summarizes the medical history of the patient from the initial note through discharge, including test results, medications, and any other information included in this section in the initial note.

Subjective (S)

The Subjective section of the Discharge Notes includes updates or additional information regarding the patient's status since the most recent note was written, *or* completely summarizes the history of the patient from the initial note through discharge, whether the patient feels the goals set were achieved, and whether the patient feels ready to function at home or work.

Objective (O)
Systems Review

The Systems Review is either not mentioned at all in the Discharge Note, or completely summarizes the Systems Review written in the initial note.

Reporting of Tests and Measures

The Discharge Summary updates the patient's status since the last note was written, or completely summarizes the patient's condition upon discharge from the facility (more similar to the initial note in format and length).

Assessment (A)
Evaluation

Evaluation may include the following:

1. A discussion of any remaining functional limitations
2. A discussion of suggested further therapy
3. A discussion of whether or not the patient achieved the Expected Outcomes and Anticipated Goals
4. Referrals made to other health professionals

Diagnosis

Diagnosis may include a discussion of the progression of the patient through diagnostic categories or movement dysfunction diagnoses, *or* a diagnosis section similar to the initial note.

Prognosis

Prognosis may include a prognosis for meeting an Expected Outcome that will be met when the patient completes all therapy for this episode of care.

Plan of Care (P)
Expected Outcomes

The discharge summary indicates which of the Expected Outcomes have been achieved and which have not (and why not).

Anticipated Goals

In some facilities, comments are made on the most recently set Anticipated Goals and why they were or were not achieved. In other facilities, no comment is made on the Anticipated Goals.

Intervention Plan

The following information should be briefly stated:

1. Interventions delivered
2. If instruction in a home program was done and the patient's or caregiver's level of independence in the program
3. If any other type of instruction of the patient or family was performed and the level of learning that occurred (in observable terms)
4. If the patient was sold any type of equipment
5. If written instructions for any equipment sold to the patient were given
6. The number of times the patient was seen in therapy
7. Any instances of the patient skipping or canceling treatment sessions
8. If and when the patient was not seen or was put on hold and why
9. To where the patient was discharged
10. The reason for discharge from PT
11. Recommendations for follow-up interventions or care given to the patient

Bibliography

1. American Physical Therapy Association: Guide to Physical Therapist Practice, ed. 2, and CD-ROM. American Physical Therapy Association, Alexandria, VA, 2003.

2. Defensible Documentation for Patient/Client Management. Accessed at http://www.apta.org/AM/Template.cfm?Section=Documentation4&Template=/MembersOnly.cfm&ContentID= 37776 on March 9, 2007.

3. American Physical Therapy Association: Guidelines: Physical Therapy Documentation of Patient/Client Management. Accessed at http://www.apta.org/AM/Template.cfm?Section=Home&TEMPLATE=/CM/ ContentDisplay.cfm&CONTENTID=31688 on March 9, 2007.

D Tips for Note Writing for Third-Party Payors

Examination

1. The current medical diagnosis and any relevant secondary medical diagnoses or test results should be included. At times, the relevant secondary medical diagnosis can help justify the need for examination of a patient's functional level, even if the patient does not need prolonged OT or PT.

2. The onset of the current medical diagnosis and the date that therapy began are essential to the D/C note.

3. *Do not* list irrelevant information. Information from the patient or significant others should help demonstrate the need for therapy.

4. When you report any complaints, keep the complaints brief and to the point. What does the patient see as his or her biggest problem? How does this problem tie into patient function (if the problem itself is not functional)?

5. Have the patient rate his or her complaints on a scale. Use of a pain scale is one example. Functional abilities at home and the amount of assistance the patient required to do them (e.g., the number of people needed) is another. Subjective information put on a type of scale can be used to re-evaluate the patient's progress. Use a quality-of-life scale if at all possible.

6. Avoid listing nonspecific complaints in progress notes that are the result of normal patient discouragement. Statements like "I don't think I'm doing very well" may serve as a red flag to the reviewers and may not be validated by the results of tests and measures.

7. *Do* list the patient's level of functioning prior to the onset of his or her current diagnosis. This can help justify the need for therapy in the case of a chronic illness. It can also justify the need for teaching by the therapist. (For example, a patient who has never used a walker before needs instruction in its proper use.)

8. *Do* briefly describe the patient's living environment, social history, and employment status and environment. Does the patient live alone? Who will be home during the day to care for the patient, if needed? Are there steps present, and is there a handrail? Are the steps essential for the patient to ambulate? What is the distance from the bed to the bathroom, to the kitchen, and so forth? Are the surfaces on the floors carpeted, tiled, linoleum, or hardwood, and are there any throw rugs present? Are there grab bars in the bathroom around the toilet or tub? Can a wheelchair fit through the doorways and turn in the rooms?

9. Briefly list any relevant history from the patient under the appropriate subcategories. Has the patient's functional status declined recently and why? Include whether the patient has received therapy before, why, and when. Also, has the patient ever used an assistive device before? Why and when? Does the patient own an assistive device or adaptive equipment?

10. Find out the patient's goals. What are the patient's plans upon discharge from therapy? What does he or she want to be able to do upon discharge from therapy that he or she cannot do at its initiation?

11. Measure *everything;* avoid estimates and/or terms like "appears" or "functional." All items should be quantified initially to show progress when re-examined later.

12. Show deficits that require a therapist's skilled care versus that of an aide/technician or family member. For example, show how your instruction is necessary, examine the speed of transfer and the movement of each body part during transfers, as well as the assistance needed. Only a PT or OT can work on deviations; an aide can work on mere distance and assistance.

13. Be sure to put a baseline measurement of an activity or deficit in your note if you plan an outcome or an intervention that includes that activity.

14. Show significant functional deficits and how tests and measures relate to them.

15. Be careful when reporting mental status. If you are in doubt of a patient's cognitive status, do not guess and do not emphasize the negative. A patient may be a little confused, but he or she may still be able to follow commands well and gain much benefit from therapy. Avoid terms such as *confused.* If a patient is disoriented to the date, but is oriented to person, place, and task, be specific in what you state. Emphasize the patient's ability to participate in therapy.

16. Use evidence-based tests and measures, if possible.

17. Do not forget to take vital signs. Gait or transfer training for the sake of endurance is not reimbursable because an aide can ambulate a patient who needs only standby assistance but needs to increase ambulation distance. However, if the heart rate, blood pressure, or respiratory rate increases abnormally

during ambulation, a therapist's level of skill is needed to further train the patient in ambulation.

18. Re-examine on a regular basis. It is easier to reset goals and assess the effectiveness of interventions if consistent data are available on a regular basis.

Evaluation

1. Explain why a patient's progress may be slower than the usual progress made by patients with the same diagnosis.
2. Explain how impairments relate to function.
3. Explain the rationale for your Plan of Care. Be sure that you explain why the services of a physical therapist are needed instead of the services of a nurse aide or personal assistant for the patient.

Plan of Care

1. Use a specific time estimate for achieving your goals. If goals are not met within an estimated time, explain why, and reset your goals.
2. Expected Outcomes and Anticipated Goals should:
   a. Focus on *the patient* and what he or she will be able to do.
   b. State *the specific behavior* the patient will exhibit.
   c. State any *special conditions* or *equipment* needed or used: assistive devices, weight-bearing status, type of wraps, prosthetics, orthotics, w/c, and so forth.
   d. Be *measurable, tied to functional activities,* and *include time frames* in which they will be achieved.

3. Be sure you continue to justify the need for skilled therapy as you near the completion of expected outcomes.
4. Point out progress that the patient has made toward the Expected Outcomes and Anticipated Goals as well as further goals.
5. Include the frequency with which the patient is seen.
6. Be specific enough to describe the interventions that require a therapist versus an aide.
7. Justify the amount of time you spend with the patient by stating the type and amount of each intervention the patient receives.

Other

1. Make sure that all forms required by third-party payors are complete and that the information required is in the appropriate section and is clear, concise, and easy to find.
2. Attach all notes required by third-party payors. Keep yourself updated on the frequency of note writing required. Save yourself time by not writing progress notes any more frequently than required; progress is easier to see over a longer period.
3. For third-party payors who require preauthorization for therapy, make sure you have preauthorization and a preauthorization number if the organization issues one. Do not exceed the number of preauthorized therapy sessions until and unless you obtain preauthorization for more therapy. Be proactive: Advocate for your patient and his or her best interests with respect to third-party payors.

Bibliography

1. American Physical Therapy Association: Guide to Physical Therapist Practice, ed. 2, and CD-ROM. American Physical Therapy Association, Alexandria, VA, 2003.
2. Defensible Documentation for Patient/Client Management. Accessed at http://www.apta.org/AM/Template.cfm?Section=Documentation4&Template=/MembersOnly.cfm&ContentID=37776 on March 9, 2007.
3. American Physical Therapy Association: Guidelines: Physical Therapy Documentation of Patient/Client Management. Accessed at http://www.apta.org/AM/Template.cfm? Section=Home&TEMPLATE=/CM/ ContentDisplay.cfm& CONTENTID= 31688 on March 9, 2007.